Swine Production and Management

THE AUTHOR

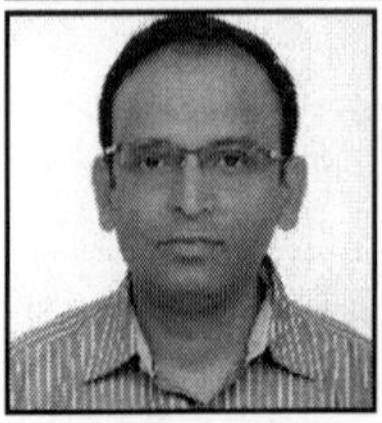

Dr. Niraj Kumar is Professor of Animal Genetics & Breeding working in College of Veterinary Medicine, Mekelle University, Mekelle since 2010. He has worked as Veterinary Doctor in several Middle East and African countries. He has published 2 books and more than 60 research publications from nationally and internationally acclaimed publishing houses/journals.

Swine Production and Management

– Edited by –

Dr. Niraj Kumar

– Contributors –

Dr. Niraj Kumar • Dr. Berihu Gebrekidan Teklehaymanot • Tsegay Tkue • Dr. Awot Teklu Mebratu • Dr. Abrha Bsrat Hailu • Dr. Etsay Kebede Assefa • Dr. Yohannes T. Asfaw • Dr. Gebregiorgis Ashebir Gebereselassie • Dr. Nigus Abebe Shumuye • Dr. Endale Balcha Gurmu • Dr. Muuz Gebru Sahle • Dr. Kiros Abebe • Mr. Hailay Kidanu • Dr. Merhawit Reda Kidane

2022

Daya Publishing House®
A Division of
Astral International Pvt. Ltd.
New Delhi – 110 002

ISBN: 978-93-5461-389-0 (HB)

Published by : **Daya Publishing House®**
A Division of
Astral International Pvt. Ltd.
– ISO 9001:2015 Certified Company –
4736/23, Ansari Road, Darya Ganj
New Delhi-110 002
Ph. 011-43549197, 8130496929
E-mail: info@astralint.com
Website: www.astralint.com

Digitally Printed at : Replika Press Pvt. Ltd.

Preface

This book on Swine Production and Management emphasizes the swine rearing in totality. The authors have provided a technical basis for the successful raising of swine in both temperate and tropical environments. Pork is consumed the most than any other terrestrial meat and the competitive position of pork as a food source both in the developed and developing countries have continued to be strengthened during the past few decades. This book contains a classic guide to swine farming that presents the reader with all the fundamental information they would need to know about breeding and farming pigs.

This book is written in simple language and it deals with the basic principles of the establishment of a new swine farm, its management, good practices and ideal conditions for optimum production of the pig. Besides production and management, this book also contains marketing, the economics of production, and important diseases of pigs. Considering the importance of swine in the field of veterinary and animal sciences, this book has been written to provide a more academic, scientific and field-oriented approach, thus making it suitable to the needs of academicians, scientists, students, field practitioners and the general reader.

Niraj et al.

Contents

The Contributor's

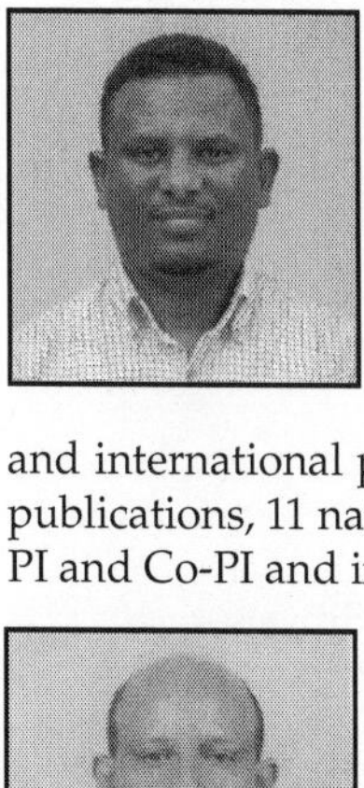

Dr. Berihu Gebrekidan Teklehaymanot is an Associate Professor in Department of Veterinary Theriogenology and Welfare, College of Veterinary Sciences, Mekelle University, Ethiopia. His current research and development interest focuses on animal health, animal biotechnology and animal reproduction. Since last 13 years, he served in the university in different level of leadership including his 6 years of deanship. He also served as a chairperson for National Veterinary Education Forum, in Ethiopia for 4 years. He worked with national and international partners on livestock development and one health approach. He has 37 publications, 11 national and international awards and recognitions, 17 different projects as PI and Co-PI and in many national and regional level committee memberships.

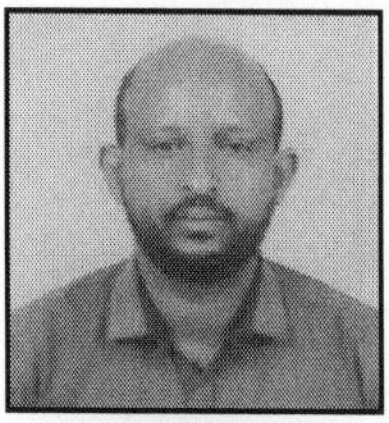

Mr. Tsegay Tkue Gebrewahd is an Associate Professor in the department of veterinary Theriogenology and welfare, college of veterinary sciences, Mekelle University since 2008. He has published 25 research articles in reputable peer-reviewed national and international journals. Moreover, he has prepared two teaching materials (Principles of Animal Genetics and Breeding and poultry and swine production) for undergraduate DVM students. Currently, he is the livestock farms center coordination office head in the college of veterinary sciences, Mekelle University.

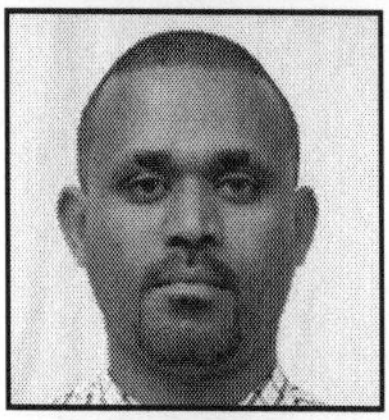

Dr. Awot Teklu Mebratu (DVM, MSc, PhD candidate) is an Associate Professor at Mekelle University, College of Veterinary Sciences, Department of Theriogenology and Welfare. Since his recruitment in 2008, Dr. Awot has a teaching and research experience of 12 years at different sectors in the University. So far, he has published 22 research articles and prepared a teaching material in his institution.

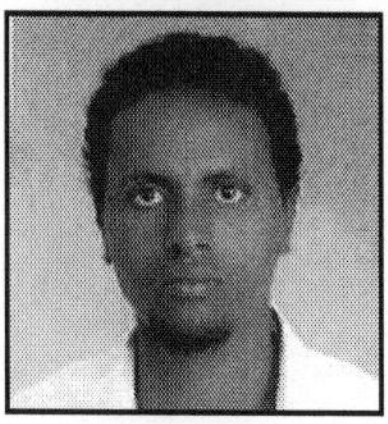

Dr. Abrha Bsrat Hailu is Associate Professor of working in College of Veterinary Medicine, Mekelle University, Mekelle. He completed his MSc on Tropical and Infectious Disease at Aklilu Lemma Institute of Pathobiology (graduated in 2012) with a project on "Molecular Epidemiology of Cutaneous Leishmaniosis in Human". He participate in various conferences, training and exchange programs in different countries (Italy, USA, China, South Africa, Senegal, Uganda, Kenya, and Ethiopia). He has published more than 25 research publications from nationally and internationally acclaimed publishing houses/journals.

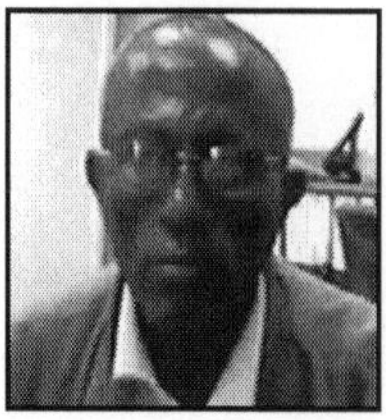

Dr. Etsay Kebede Assefa had been contributing in Mekelle University College of Dryland Agriculture in Department of Animal Science and Faculty of Veterinary Medicine as guest instructor from 2000- 2005. He worked in formerly named Faculty of Veterinary Medicine and now in the College of Veterinary Sciences as Associate Professor since 2006. He published 32 articles, one book and translated manual of syndromic surveillance from English to two local languages. Before joining Mekelle University, he had been working on several positions as veterinary zonal officer, fourth livestock development project coordinator, Pan African Rinderpest campaign regional coordinator, Department Head of Animal Resources and Fishery, Regional Veterinary Laboratory Head and Manager of Abergelle International Development PLC.

Dr. Yohannes Tekle Asfaw is an academic staff in Mekelle University College of Veterinary Sciences, Department of Veterinary Basics and Diagnostic Sciences, veterinary Pathology team. He is a trained veterinary Pathologist who received his MVSc from the Indian Veterinary Research Institute (IVRI) in 2010. He also is on his final year to complete his PhD study on Tropical and Infectious Diseases. He served in the college for about 12 years and during his 12 years of professional services, he taught different pathology courses including swine pathology and necropsy techniques to undergraduate and postgraduate students. On daily basis, he performs different necropsies of different animals. Moreover, he got involved in several research and consultancy projects among which he participated in swine parasitic diseases research project which is a published work. Till now, he published about 30 papers in reputable journals, and he co-authored a manual disease syndrome. He also prepared different training manuals on Disease prevention and control in different food animals.

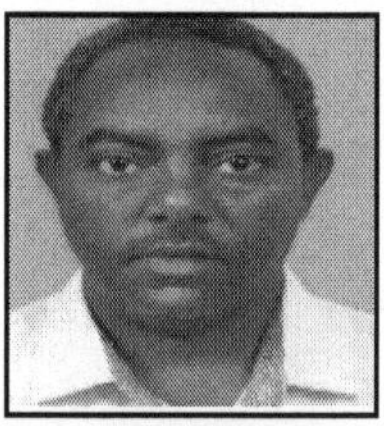

Dr. Gebregiorgis Ashebir Gebereselassie is an Associate Professor of Animal Reproduction, Gynecology and Obstetrics in College of Veterinary Sciences, Mekelle University. He served 8 years as field veterinarian and 14 year as University Instructor and researcher. He published more than 20 research articles in peer reviewed journals. Now served as Head of the Department of Theriogenology and Welfare.

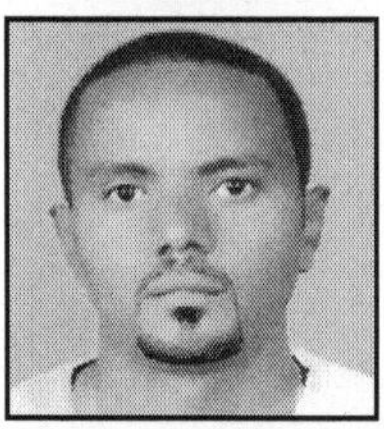

Dr. Endale Balcha Gurmu is an Associate Professor in Department of Veterinary Public Health and food safety, College of Veterinary Sciences, Mekelle University. He has over 13 years of teaching experience and supervised over 40 undergraduate and postgraduate students. He published around 14 research articles in peer reviewed journals. The author has also been in a number of community engagements with regard to food hygiene and safety.

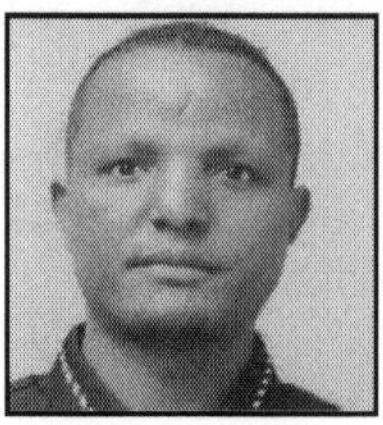

Dr. Nigus Abebe Shumuye is an Assistant Professor in Tropical and Infectious Diseases working at the department of Veterinary Clinical Medicine and Epidemiology, CVS, MU since July 2005. Currently, he is PhD candidate in China. He published more than 15 articles in peer reviewed journals.

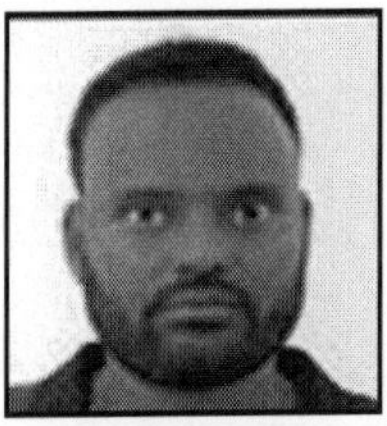

Dr. Muuz Gebru Sahle is an Associate Professor in the Department of Veterinary Basic and Diagnostic Sciences in College of Veterinary Sciences, Mekelle University. He has work experience of 11 years being engaged at teaching (under and post graduate programs), research and community service activities. He has published 19 papers and is a founding member of the Ethiopian Society for Microbiology, member of professional associations including Ethiopian Veterinary Association and American Society for Microbiology.

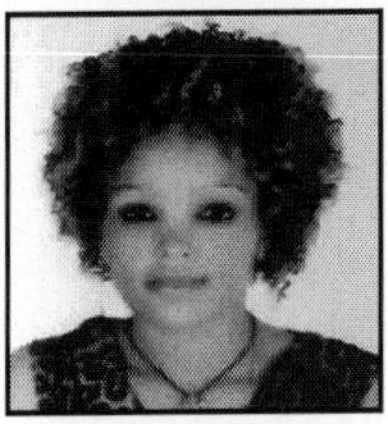

Kiros Abebe (PhD) is an Assistant Professor in Animal Production in Veterinary Theriogenology and Welfare team of College of Veterinary Sciences, Mekelle University. She has four years of experience in teaching, research and community service. She published 2 books and 9 research papers in peer reviewed journals.

Hailay Kidanu has been involved in teaching and research at the Department of Veterinary Theriogenology and Welfare, College of Veterinary Sciences, Mekelle University. He did his MSc in Animal Health and has more than 6 years of experience. He has three publication. Currently, he is working as HIV/AIDS and Reproductive health Office Coordinator at the college level.

Dr. Merhawit Reda Kidane is an Assistant Professor in the department of Veterinary Surgery and Anatomy of the College of Veterinary Sciences, Mekelle Universitysince 2017. She served as a clinician in the Teaching Hospital, College of Veterinary Sciences, Mekelle University for five years. She has participated in various research and community engagement projects as PI and Co-PI. She has published several articles in reputable journals. She has served the college in various positional assignments such as gender officer and currently working as Head of the Department of Veterinary Surgery and Anatomy, College of Veterinary Sciences, Mekelle University.

Chapter 1

Introduction

— **Dr. Niraj Kumar**

In general usage, swine are referred to as hogs and pigs. The term 'hogs' generally used for adult animals, and 'pigs' to young animals. The social and adaptable nature and omnivorous diet of the wild boar allowed early humans to domesticate it much earlier than many other forms of livestock, such as cattle. Unlike most other hoofed mammals, pigs do not have multi-chambered ruminating stomachs and cannot survive on leaves and grasses alone. Instead, they are omnivores, which means that they consume both plants and animals and that makes swine enterprises more profitable as compared to other livestock enterprises. They eat a wide variety of foods, including corns and other seeds, green vegetation, roots, tubers, fungi, fruit, eggs, insects, and small animals like snakes. In commercial/intensive system, pigs are fed mostly soybean meal and corn with a mixture of minerals and vitamins added to the diet. Forages are mostly added in gestating sows, but growing-finishing pigs can also utilize pastures, ground legume hays/meals, and others. Pigs can utilize the garbage, bakery wastes, unmarketable grains, vegetables, fruits, etc., which are not suitable for humans. The one-fourth of food grain supply in the world is lost or wasted because of weather, poor harvesting, storage, handling, etc., which can be utilized by pigs. Swine are also scavengers and can make productive use of many materials that would otherwise be wasted.

Pigs can be raised in different styles of farming. Intensive commercial units, commercial free-range enterprises, extensive farming which allowed to wander around a village, town or city, or tethered in a simple shelter or kept in a pen outside the owner's house. Historically pigs were closely associated with the residence of the owner and kept in small numbers. They were considered as a source of pork, lard, and for the ability to turn food waste into meat, and often fed household kitchen waste if kept on a homestead. In developed countries, commercial/intensive farms house thousands of pigs in climate-controlled buildings. The farm activities on a pig farm depend on the types of pig husbandry. In a backyard free-ranging system where very little intervention is made by the owner and pigs are allowed to roam villages or towns and dispose of garbage. While in intensive systems where the pigs are contained in a building for the majority of their lives. Each pig farm will adapt and fit their practices to their specific situation to the local conditions and food supplies. Climate is not generally a limiting factor except where it threatens feed supply. Swine are raised in both warm and temperate climates, although young pigs must be kept warm, and sheltered from weather extremes.

Swine production provides red meat for the human diet, uses less feed than is required to produce beef or lamb, and is also a source of hides and cooking fat. The meat of swine is commonly referred to as pork, which is light red before it is cooked. White fat (lard) covers much of the swine carcass and some fat is also dispersed throughout the meat. Other food products made from pigs include bacon, pork sausage (casings made from the intestines), ham, gammon, and pork scratching (cracklings or rinds). The head of a pig can be used to make head cheese (sometimes known as brawn) which is a preserved jelly. Liver, chitterlings, blood (for blood pudding or black pudding), and other offal from pigs are also widely used for food. The skin of pig is used to produce apparel, pork rinds, seat covers, and other items. Pork is one of the most popular forms of meat for human consumption, accounting for 37% of worldwide meat production.

Pigs & humans are very similar in dental characteristics, renal morphology and physiology, eye structure and visual acuity, skin morphology and physiology, cardiovascular anatomy and physiology, digestive anatomy and physiology, etc. that is why pigs have been used commonly for biomedical research on nutrition, cardiovascular physiology, obesity, stress, dermatology, toxicology, immunology, behavior, renal physiology, experimental surgery, gastroenteritis, diabetes, drug metabolism, etc.

Pigs are currently thought to be the best source for organ donation because they are easily available and their organs are anatomically comparable in size. Also, new infectious agents are less likely as they are domesticated for many generations and living in close association with the human. Other byproducts of pigs have been used for humans are skin, insulin, heart valves, other hormones, many enzymes, neurotransmitters, blood transfusion, and others. Specially selected and treated pigskin is used in treating massive burns. Insulin from pigs is chemically very similar to that of humans, thus being used to treat diabetics. Heart valves are specially preserved and treated valves are surgically implanted in humans since 1971.

The relatively short, stiff, coarse hairs of the pig are called bristles and are commonly used as paintbrushes. Solid or liquid excretory wastes form pig farms can be used to fertilize crop fields. Because of their foraging abilities and excellent sense of smell, they are used to find truffles (a kind of mushroom) in many European countries. Both wild and feral pigs are commonly hunted. Some breeds of pig are kept as pets i.e. the Asian pot-bellied pig.

Pigs have a binocular vision of 35 to 50 and a panoramic vision of approximately 310 . Like sheep, they have no eye accommodation and lift their heads to see distant objects. The extent to which pigs have the color vision is still not clear but the presence of cone cells in the retina with two distinct wavelength sensitivities for blue and green, suggests that at least some color vision is present.

Pigs have a well-developed sense of smell. Rather vision, olfactory stimuli are used in the identification of other pigs. Hearing is also well developed, and localization of sounds is made by moving the head. Pigs use auditory stimuli extensively as a means of communication in all social activities. Alarm or aversive stimuli are transmitted to other pigs not only by auditory cues but also by pheromones. Similarly, the identification between the sow and her piglets is by vocal cues and olfactory.

The only places where swine production is not suitable are where religious law (as in Islam and Orthodox Judaism, for example) or strong tradition forbids the consumption of pork. Pigs intersect with religion and culture in several ways. Considering the pig to be an unclean animal, in Judaism and Islam, it is forbidden to consume swine or pork in any form. In Christianity, pigs are allied with Saint Anthony, the patron saint of swine herds. In Hinduism, God Vishnu took the form of a boar to save the earth from a demon that had dragged it to the bottom of the sea.

Summarily, swine production has many advantages. Swine convert feed to meat more efficiently than cattle or sheep do. A beef steer requires about nine pounds of feed to produce a pound of beef, a lamb requires about eight pounds, while a hog requires from four to five pounds of feed per pound of live weight. Swine are productive, generally producing two farrows per year and from six to twelve piglets per litter. Swine yield more useable carcass compared to other animals that produce red meat. Dressing yield is from 65 to 80 percent for swine, but 50 to 60 percent for cattle, and 45 to 55 percent for sheep and lambs. Pigs can convert inedible wastes and by-products into the meat. Garbage such as food and garden scraps are usually cooked before being fed to hogs to prevent the spread of disease. Very little labor is required in swine farming. It is possible to get by with a small investment for buildings and equipment. Returns come quickly. A gilt (young female swine) may be bred at eight months, and the pigs are ready for slaughter six months after farrowing. Hogs are an excellent source of home-processed meats. This is due to the superior curing, ease of dressing and, keeping qualities of pork.

1.1 Taxonomical Classification of the Pig

Kingdom:	Animalia
Phylum:	Chordata
Subphylum:	Vertebrata
Class:	Mammalia
Subclass:	Utheria
Order:	Artiodactyla
Family:	Suidae
Genus:	Sus Linn.
Species:	S. scrofa (wild boar)
	S. domesticus (domestic pig)
Synonyms:	Sus scrofa domestica; Sus domesticus; Sus domestica

Pigs are even-toed ungulate mammals of the order Artiodactyla and the genus Sus, within the Suidae family. They are native to Eurasia and northern Africa. The domestic pig, Sus scrofa domesticus, was one of the first animals domesticated by humans from its ancestor, the common Eurasian wild boar (Sus scrofa), and is still today one of the most important domestic animals. The domestic pig is considered to be a subspecies of the wild boar and given name Sus scrofa by Carl Linnaeus in 1758. After that, the formal name of the domestic pig is Sus scrofa domesticus. However, in 1777, Johann Christian Polycarp Erxleben classified the domestic pig as a separate species and gave e name Sus domesticus, which is still used by some taxonomists.

Historical data indicates the pig was domesticated by 4900 B.C. in China, and pigs were raised in Europe as early as 1500 B.C. Pigs were first introduced into North America by Hernado de Soto in 1539, with further introductions into Mexico by Hernando Cortez in 1600. Untamed pigs can be found in every continent except Australia, as well as in most temperate islands in both hemispheres. The principal varieties were enlisted as:

1. European Wild Boar (Sus Scrofa) - From Europe to Central Asia, from the Baltic to North Africa, as well as in some parts of North America.
2. Asiatic Wild Boar (Sus scrofa cristatus; subspecies) Ceylon (Sri Lanka), India, Siam (Thailand), China, and various areas within that general region.
3. Others - Wart Hog, Collared Peccaries, Babirussa, etc.

All breeds of domestic pigs were originally descended from Sus scrofa. They can mate successfully to produce offspring with Wild Boar. In addition to the modern breeds of swine, there are many indigenous species of swine throughout the world including Sus ahoenobarbus (Palawan bearded pig), Sus bucculentus (Vietnam warty pig), Sus oliveri (Mindoro warty pig), Sus salvanius (the Pygmy Hog), Sus verrucosus (the Javan Warty Pig), Sus barbatus (the Bearded Pig), Sus celebensis (the Sulawesi Warty Pig), Sus philippensis (the Philippine Warty Pig) and Sus cebifrons (The Visayan Warty Pig). Several extinct species are known from fossils which are Sus australis (early Pleistocene of China), Sus bijiashanensis (early Pleistocene of China), Sus falconeri (Pleistocene of the Siwalik region, India), Sus houi (Pleistocene of China), Sus hysudricus, Sus jiaoshanensis (early Pleistocene of China), Sus liuchengensis (early Pleistocene of China), Sus lydekkeri(Pleistocene of China), Sus offecinalis (China), Sus peii (early Pleistocene of China), Sus subtriquetra, Sus strozzi and Sus xiaozhu (early Pleistocene of China).

1.2 Geographic Distribution

Swine is distributed across the world. The estimated global swine population is around 978 million live heads in 2018 (FAOSTAT, 2018). The trend of swine production from 1994 to 2018 is shown in figure 1.1. The estimated global swine inventory was over 883 million in 1994 and over 898 million in 2000 shows an increasing trend for the last two decades. The countries of Asia have the largest inventory of swine in the world, accounting for 58.7% of the total global inventory.

The countries of the European Union account for nearly 20.9% of the global inventory, followed by North America with over 16.9% in 2018 (table 1.1, figure 1.1 and 1.2).

Table 1.1: Swine Population (Continent wise)

Area	*Population (live heads)*	*Percent of world population*
Africa	27120166.04	2.9%
Americas	157019594	16.9%
Asia	545002289.8	58.7%
Europe	194618090.1	20.9%
Oceania	5381616.76	0.6%
World total	978332119	100.00

Source: FAOSTAT, 2018

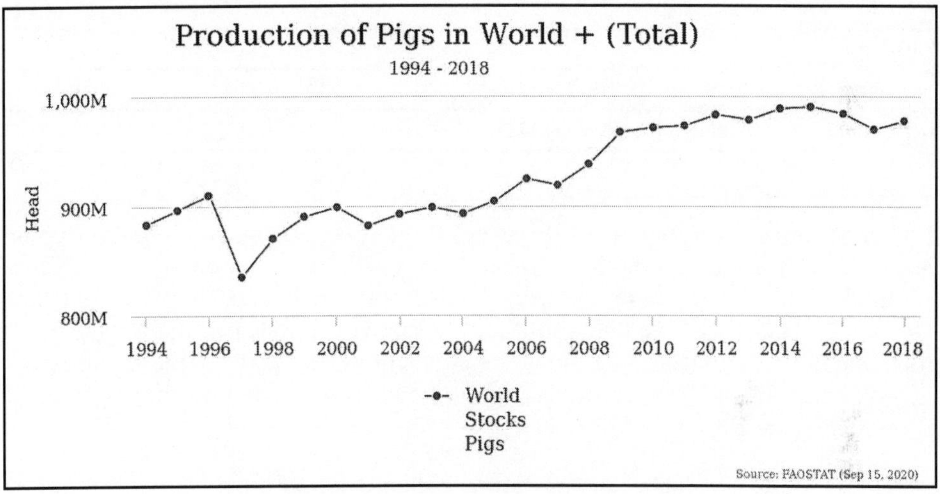

Figure 1.1: Production of pigs in the world (1994-2018)

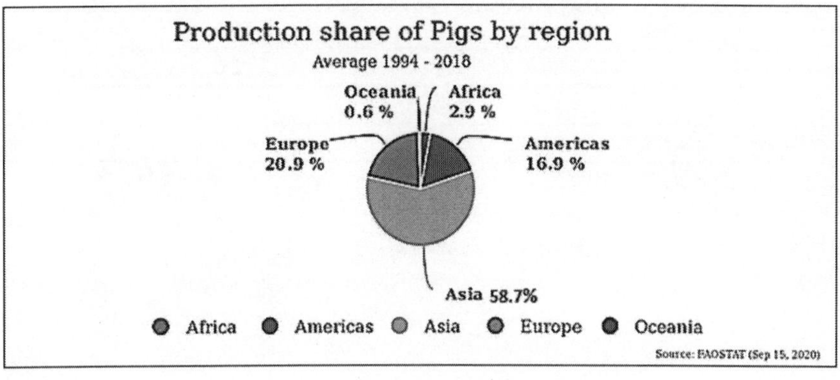

Figure 1.2: Production share of Pigs by region.

The Peoples Republic of China has the highest number of swine in the world, with an estimated inventory of 436 million pigs or approximately 44.59% of the global total in 2018 (table 1.2).

Table 1.2: Swine inventory in selected countries in 2018

Area	*Population (live heads)*	*Percent of the world population*
China, mainland	436335684.6	44.59
United States of America	63682620	6.50
Brazil	35472845.92	3.62
Germany	26400596.24	2.69
Viet Nam	24375059.96	2.49
Spain	24046994.6	2.45
Russian Federation	18632038.52	1.90
Mexico	15834782.84	1.61
Myanmar	15710120.24	1.60
France	14283109.92	1.45

1.3 Pork consumption pattern

Food outlook (FAO, 2013) data revealed that pork is consumed the most than any other terrestrial meat (table 1.3). About 37% of all meat consumed in the world is pork (110 million metric tonnes, mmt) which is ahead of beef (67 mmt) and chicken (104 mmt). In 2011, China had about half of the world pork production (50 mmt) followed by the USA (10 mmt) and Germany (5 mmt). Over 80% of the world's pork is produced in Asia, North America, and the EU. The production share of meat is shown in figure 1.3.

Table 1.3: Pork consumption in the world.

Meat	Meat consumed, 2012 (mmt)	Percentage of Meat (%)
Pork/Porcine	110.8	37.4
Poultry	104.5	35.3
Bovine	66.8	22.6
Ovine	13.9	4.7
Total common meat	296.0	100.0

Source: Food outlook, FAO, 2013

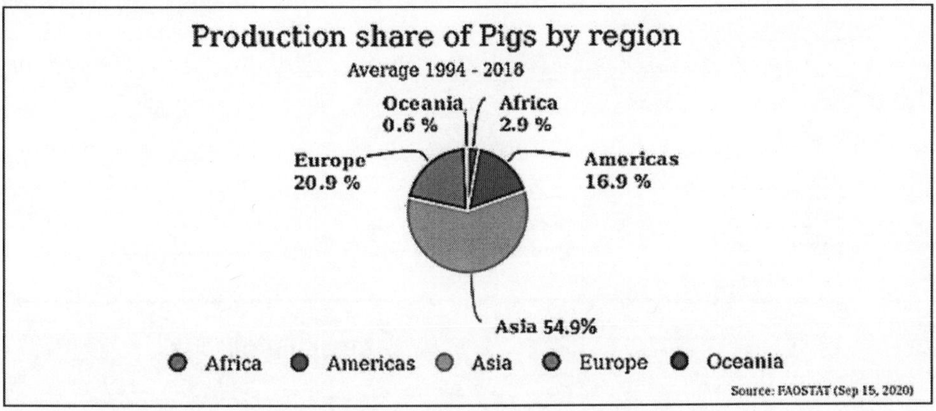

Figure 1.3: Production share of Meat, pig by region.

□□□

Chapter 2

General Body Features and Handling of Pigs

— Dr. Niraj Kumar

It is important to know body parts of a pig (figure 2.1) as it is useful while studying breed characteristics, judging animals, handling, recording physiological parameters (like body temperature, pulse rate, respiration rate, and collection of blood), locating external injury or abnormalities on the body, writing reports of treatments and classification of pigs.

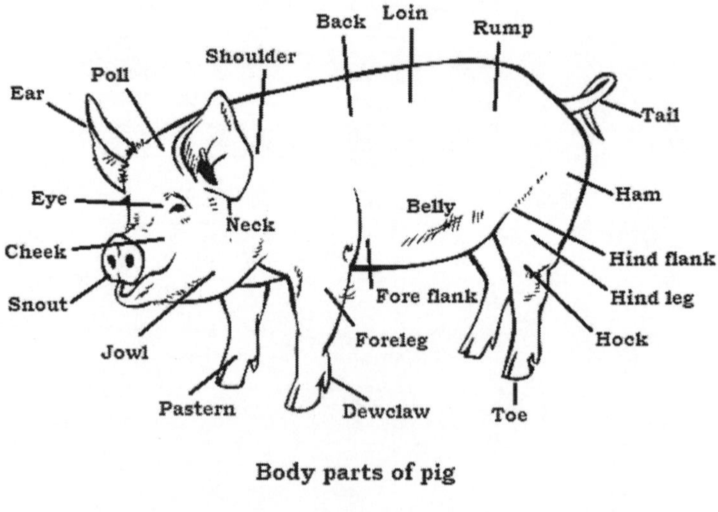

Figure 2.1: Body parts of pig

A typical pig has a large head with a long snout which is strengthened by a special pre-nasal bone and by a disk of cartilage at the tip (figure 2.2). The snout is an acute sense organ and very useful for digging soil while searching feed. Each trotter (foot) has four hooves (toes). The two larger central toes are used to bears most of the body weight and the outer two are used for grip in soft ground (figure 2.3).

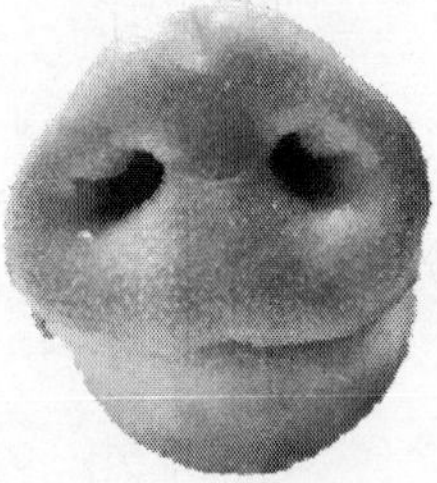

Figure 2.2: Disk of cartilage at the tip of snout.

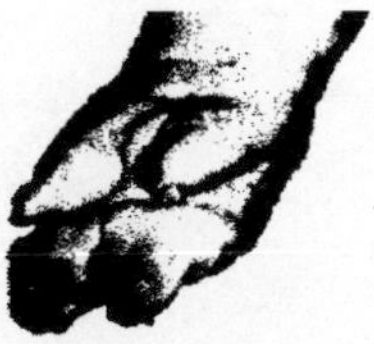

Figure 2.3: Four hoofed toes of pig.

The number of teeth in the upper and lower jaw of the pig is 44 (table 2.1). The rear teeth are adapted for crushing. Canine teeth in males form tusks that grow continuously.

Table 2.1: Dentition in pigs

Jaw	*Incisors*	*Canines*	*Premolars*	*Molars*	*Total*	*Grand total*
Upper	3+3	1+1	4+4	3+3	22	44
Jaw	3+3	1+1	4+4	3+3	22	

The eruption of all temporary teeth is completed by five months of age. The eruption of teeth will indicate the age of the pig (table 2.2).

Table 2.2: Age of Eruption of permanent teeth in pigs

Eruption of permanent teeth	*Age of pig*
First pair corner incisors	6 months of age
Second pair lateral incisors	10 months of age
Third pair middle incisors	12 months of age
Fourth pair central incisors	18 months of age

Pigs have extremely rugged skeletons (figure 2.4) which support larger weight, in proportion to size, than any other farm animal.

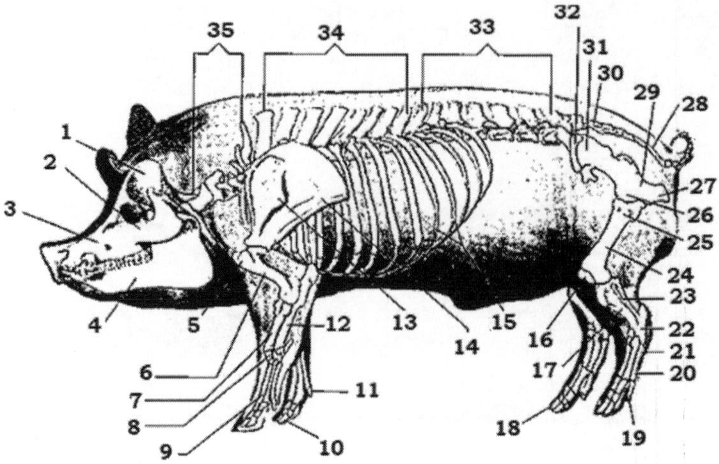

Figure: Skeletal system of pig. 1.Cranium, 2.Zygomatic arch, 3.Facial region, 4.Mandible, 5.Manubrium of sternum, 6.Humerus, 7.Radius, 8.Carpals, 9.Metacarpals, 10.Main phalanges, 11.Accessory phalanges, 12.Ulna, 13.Scapular spine, 14.Scapula, 15.Ribs, 16.Patella, 17.Tibia, 18.Main Phalanges, 19.Accessory phalanges, 20.metatarsals, 21.Tarsals, 22.Calcaneus, 23.Fibula, 24.Femur, 25.Greater trochanter, 26.Pubis, 27.Ischeal tuberosity, 28.Caudal vertebrae, 29.Ischium, 30.Scarum, 31.Illium, 32.Iliac crest, 33.Lumber vertebrae, 34.Thoracic

Figure 2.4: Skeletal system of pig.

2.2 Handling and restraining pigs

Proper swine handling is an important task for physical examination and welfare. Pigs are handled by considering its behavioral principles such as point of balance and flight zone and handlers should be trained for that. While restraining or when frightened, pig usually grunts or may squeal loudly.

Pig is having a hardy appearance but cannot stand very rough handling, particularly during hot weather. If harsh force is used, pigs easily become alert and may become stubborn, loud, and even furious, particularly when handling sows with litters or older boars. Pigs should be allowed to rest when become overexcited.

Pigs are handled or restrained for close examination of the animal, teeth clipping and de-tusking, prior to anesthesia, surgical procedures, tail docking, castration, routine injections, lancing abscesses, identification of pigs, moving to a different pen or farrowing crate, blood sampling, weighing, data and sample collection. The equipment needed for moving, handling, and restraining pigs are pig handling boards, paddles, trapping crates, snare or snubbing rope, trough, and bucket. There are several methods to restraining pigs like with a noose (a loop with a running knot of rope to trap animals), sedation or, a combination of both or by using a chase board.

Flight zone

It is easy to handle pig if the flight zone is well understood. The flight zone is the personal space of pig and the size of an individual's flight zone is determined by their level of stress or excitement and their tameness. The panoramic range of vision in swine is 3100. The blind spot is directly behind the swine (light gray below) and this area should be avoided. For handling pigs, the best site for the handler is between positions A and B on the edge of the flight zone (figure 2.5).

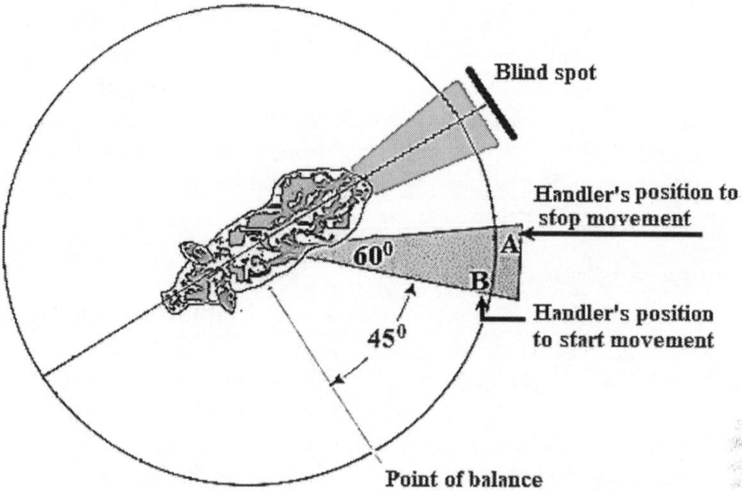

Figure 2.5: Handling pigs by flight zone.

For the forward movement of the swine, the handler should enter the flight zone behind the "point of balance" or shoulder. Work at a 45-600 angle behind the animal's shoulder, moving back and forth parallel to the direction you want the animal to move. Move toward B to start the movement. Move to A to stop the animal's movement. If a handler walks deep into the flight zone, swine will have a tendency to move in a direction opposite of the handler's movement. If the handler moves from the head toward the rear then the swine will usually move forward. If the handler move in front of the point of balance then swine will move backward. Pig becomes panic when there is a sudden, deep invasion of the flight zone.

Things to Avoid to Prevent Injury

It is important to know some common practices to avoid injury to pigs as well as handlers while handling pigs. Separating sows from piglets makes sows aggressive and care will be taken while reaching into the pen. Sudden movements in the blind spot cause the animal to panic and run away, possibly causing injury to the animal or handler. Swine become nervous when separated from the herd. Cornering will increase the stress on the animal. Patches of light and dark, air drafts, loud noises, can cause animals to panic, or hesitate or stop moving. A stressed, frightened, or excited pig may run through wire fencing, inflicting injury upon itself.

Method of Moving Pigs

Using pig behavior is an effective way to move pigs. Pigs move best when handled in a group, and when they are following a leader or at least walking side-by-side with other pigs. Overcrowded pigs cannot easily turn around. Moving people distract pigs. Use humane moving devices when moving pigs (e.g. chase boards, shakers). Pig-handling boards facilitate the movement of pigs with minimal effort when used intelligently by handlers. Animals of all ages may be moved through corridors or narrow passageways with relative ease. Pigs may hesitate and refuse to move if they encounter shadows, bright spots, a change in flooring type or texture, drains, metal grates, or flapping objects. As pigs effectively move through small openings, it is essential to keep them moving between solid barriers. They will move more readily into well-lighted areas but not into darkened ones. When a bucket is placed over a pig's head, it may move in the reverse direction. If little feed is put in the bucket and holds it in front of the animal's snout then the pig will usually follow willingly.

Restraining of Piglets

Piglets can be caught from behind and held by grasping the hind leg just above the hock. Swinging should be avoided while handling. For lifting a small piglet, one hand is placed under the chest and then the piglet is lifted. While holding the piglet the weight should be against the body of the handler. Never grab piglets by the ears or the tail. When putting piglets down, it should be kept down gently by keeping its front legs first. Piglets can also be herded using a pig sorting board, noise shakers, or and flight zone principles.

Restraining of Growing-finishing Pigs

A pig up to 50 kg can be restrained by a person standing astride it, with a leg against each shoulder, and holding on to its ears. For vaccinations, castrations, or for giving injections, pigs should be lifted by its hind legs, turned so that it faces the same direction as the handler, and gripped between the knees with its head downwards and front feet still on the floor. Pigs can be restrained in a trough, with its ventral side up. If assistants are available, they may hold the pig in the trough, or it may be held by a rope passing from one leg around the outside of the trough to a leg on the opposite side.

Restraining of Older Pigs

Boar requires extra precautions as they can be quite aggressive. Saw increases aggression during estrus or at/near farrowing. Care should be taken when sows are in their reproductive cycle and handled cautiously. An older pig generally is restrained using a nose snare, pig holder (figure 2.6), or snubbing rope (figure 2.7) placed around the upper jaw behind the canine teeth. The handler should hold the snare and stand directly in front of the pig. This causes the pig to pull back and this is quite sufficient restraint for clipping tusks, vaccinations, treating wounds, collecting a blood sample from the suborbital sinus, and oral dosing. If more complete or longer immobilization is required, a trapping crate may be used. When a pig enters the crate and jabs its nose through the opening, the handle may be pulled to tighten the opening around its neck.

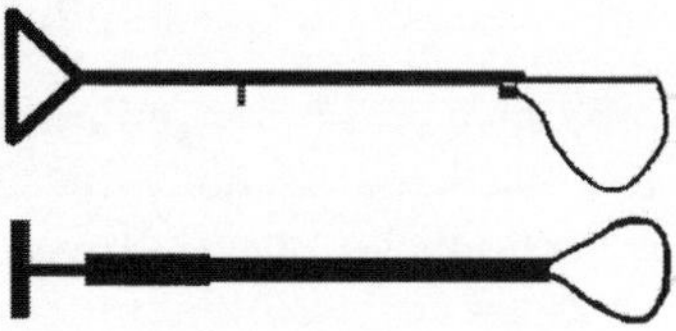

Figure 2.6: Pig holders.

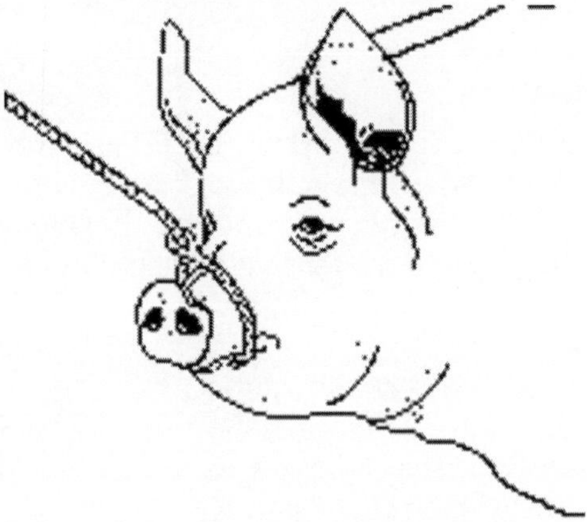

Figure 2.7: Snubbing rope.

Restraining by Sedation

This process is used for restraining pigs for long duration for surgical intervention, de-tusking boars, and lancing abscesses. This can also be used in case of aggressive or furious boars which are often a threat to handlers. Material required for this process is azaperone, acetylpromazine, or any other sedative, 10 ml syringe, 25mm to 38 mm 16g needles, a rope with a loop at both the ends, and a drum. Pigs are restrained with the rope as the handler stands by the side of the pig's shoulder. Rope is held with the two hand and pulled into the mouth behind the tusk of the upper jaw. The rope is tightened with an upward movement and pulled forward to restrain the pig. The rope is then fastened to a post, bar or ring. Then azaperone is injected intramuscular at the dose rate of 2.2 mg/kg body weight of pig. The drug is fast-acting. The peak effect is reached in 15 minutes in young animals and 30 minutes in mature animals and generally lasts for one to six hours. Azaperone can be used in pigs to prevent fighting, sedation prior to anesthesia, the examination of the feet, to prevent a gilt savaging her new piglets, to calm excitable animal, prior to the transportation or any manipulative process. Acetylpromazine is most commonly used during transportation of pigs to prevent travel sickness and occasionally used as a general sedative at a dose of 0.1 mg/kg body weight.

2.3 Casting of pigs

Hand Casting: Pigs can be cast simply by pulling their legs out from under it. A snubbing rope should be used first to hold the pig in standing posture. A second handler then reaches under its body and grasps the front and rear legs on the opposite side. When the legs are pulled under the pig towards the handler, the pig falls away in its side. Feet should be tied immediately once the pig is down. The handler may hold the feed down by kneeling on the shoulder while keeping upward pressure on the front leg. This prevents the animal from getting any legs underneath the body so it must remain to lie on its side.

Birch Method of Casting

This method can be used with pigs up to 110-120 kg, involves grasping the pig's tail with the right hand and its left hind foot with the left hand. If the pig will move, the tail should be pulled. As the pig moves, pulling down on the tail and pushing up on the leg causes the pig should be rolled over onto its back.

Rope Casting

The pig should be tied using snubbing rope. For casting pig on its right side, the snubbing rope is carried back to the left hind leg and passed circling it, above the hock, from the inside out. The end of the rope is pulled, thus pulling the hock close to the head and pushing the pig off balance. The rope should be pulled when the pig is down, and the rope end passed under the standing part to be secured by a half hitch. The pig's legs can be tied together or it can be kept down by kneeling on its shoulder while holding the front leg up.

❑❑❑

Chapter 3

Swine Production System

—Dr. Niraj Kumar

Nearly 60% of the world's pig production is in Asia with a further 36% in Europe and the USA. Pigs can be reared almost anywhere in given suitable housing and management. The pig production systems in tropics are basically low input systems where pigs rooting and roaming freely around communities, which are sold or slaughtered as per the need of the owner. Some organized farms also found around cities. In the western world, these enterprises are predominantly intensive grain-fed system where pigs are raised commercially for local consumption as well as for export. There are various pig production systems that exist around the world.

3.1 Extensive or free-range system

The free-range system is the traditional way of rearing swine in most parts of the world especially in tropics. Each family keeps a few pigs that are allowed to scavenger or wander freely and pick up food when and where they can (figure 3.1). The system needs little expenditure and management with minimum disease control. Pigs move freely around the house and surroundings, scavenging and finding most of their food themselves. They may be supplemented such as farm by-products, kitchen wastes, and others. Local breeds of pigs are highly adapted to the harsh climate and poor feed quality hence pre-dominate the free-range system. Pigs are enclosed only during night hours surrounded by a fence (made by bamboo, stick, or any locally available material) with a simple roof. Generally, least or no expenditure is done by the owner for food and veterinary services.

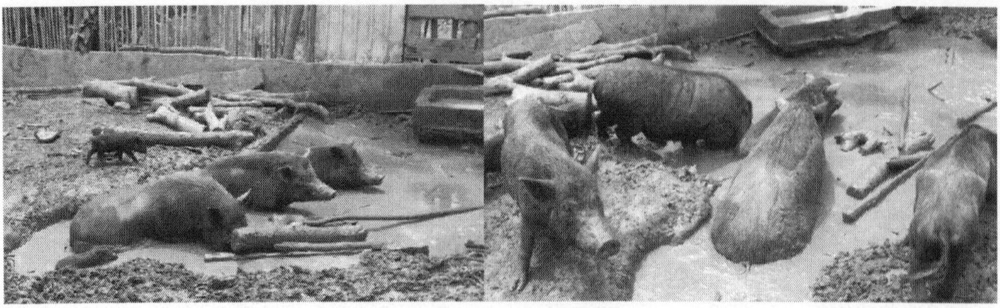

Figure 3.1: Pigs in mud under free-range scavenging system

Indigenous or local tropical breeds are more commonly maintained under this system as they are more resistant to diseases and highly adapted to hot climate. These breeds can manage with low-quality feed from kitchen wastes and search most of their food by themselves. Selection or any breeding strategies are usually not followed. Slow growth, high mortality rates in piglets, and heavy parasitic infestation are the major constraints of this system. Pigs under this system are reared not for a regular source of income or household meat consumption. They are kept as security money which is sold when extra cash needed by the owner for family.

This production system can be improved by the application of housing, feeding, and breeding management. The pigs do not grow quickly because they spend a lot of energy on their scavenging activities. The production can be improved by keeping these pig in an enclosure by providing water and feed twice a day. These animals can be raised on lower quality food by adding some supplements. Good return can be expected if special care is done for the grower, pregnant and lactating pigs. Selection and using improved boar for breeding will gradually increase the output. Parasites pose a serious problem to these pigs. A pig infested with the parasite will be in poor health and will grow very slowly. Periodic deworming and keeping pig in an enclosure will control the levels of worm infestation.

3.2 Semi- intensive pig keeping

In this system, the animals are restricted to a limited area and the farmer feeds them (figure 3.2). Once in a while, the pigs are allowed into a larger area to graze, wallow, and exercise. The animals are given fresh water and fed on kitchen wastes, food by-products, or agricultural waste once or twice a day. This system of pig keeping opens up possibilities for improved feeding and disease control, which in turn can result in faster growing and healthier pigs and larger litters. Although this system of pig keeping only requires a fairly low or medium level of financial inputs, more time and effort needs to be spent on the pigs. More technical knowledge and some level of managerial skills is required. The pigs are kept still as secured money and also to generate periodic income. Improvements to semi-intensive systems are made by focusing attention on feeding and health care practices, and by selective breeding. Housing, in particular of lactating sows and young piglets, also needs attention. Selling of manure collected in this system is also beneficial to farmers.

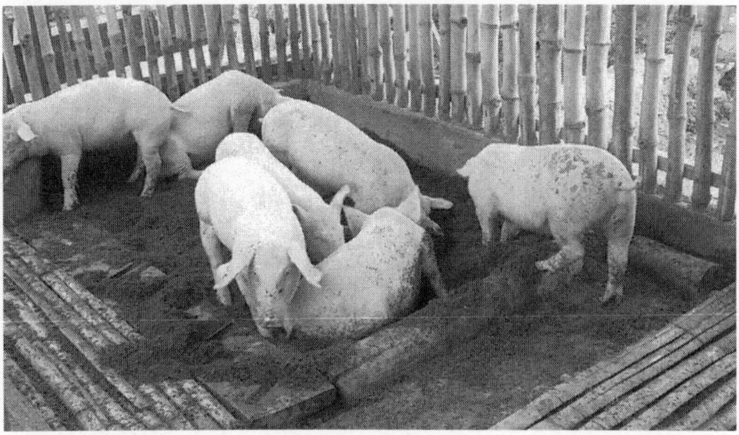

Figure 3.2: Pigs in shelter under semi- intensive system

3.3 Intensive production system

This is the commercial method of pig production. Housing is more modern and provides shade, pen space, feed, and water facilities to meet the requirements of the pigs (figure 3.3). Feeding, management, and disease control are more modern. Common breeds are exotic or crossbreds. Herd sizes may be small scale (5 Sow herd or up to 100 stock/year), medium-scale (10 Sow herd or up to 200 stock/ year), or large scale (greater than 200 stock/year).High investments are required to provide improved buildings, and to buy in feeds and medicines. Exotic or crossbred animals are kept reared by feeding commercial feed to get maximum return.

To make an intensive system economically viable requires a completely different approach to keeping pigs. The animals have to be brought to the market when they have reached the desired weight. A strategy for optimum buying and selling has to be developed, which requires the presence of regular transport and dependable sales outlets.A farmer has to decide what type of pig enterprise is most suitable for his/her circumstances. The choice of the enterprise depends on the markets, the resources available, and the motivation. Generally, there are four pig production enterprises a farmer may choose from. These enterprises are:

1. Farrow-to-finish operations: The farmer produces his own growers for a finishing operation from the sows he rears.
2. Farrow only: The farmer produces weaners from the sows he rear. He sells these weaners to other farmers.
3. Finishing operation: Farmer purchase weaners or growers and finish them for the pork market.
4. Breeding: Breeding stock production is a very specialized enterprise that is done only by the experienced pig breeders and requires heavy capital investment.

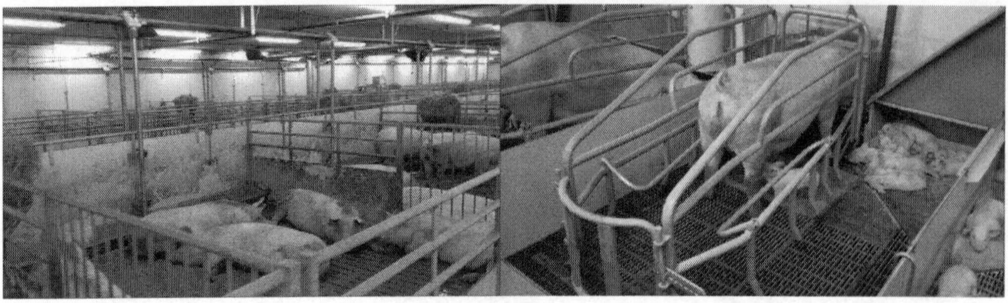

Figure 3.3: Pigs in shelter under intensive system

3.4 Pasture-based swine production system

The pasture-Based Swine production system is an alternative approach for raising swine outdoors using pasture as a major source of nutrients, particularly for gestating sows (figure 3.4). It offers the producer lower initial costs, lower production costs, and a sustainable method for producing pork. Pasture-based systems use low-cost small houses with electric fencing. As these systems require no costly buildings and handling equipment, farmers can easily reduce or expand their operation depending on prevailing market conditions. In addition, the portability of pasture systems should allow farmers to utilize the land. These systems are especially good for limited-resource and/or beginning farmers. This system has some disadvantages like it is difficult to check all the hogs and they are exposed to predators and people to steal the hogs.

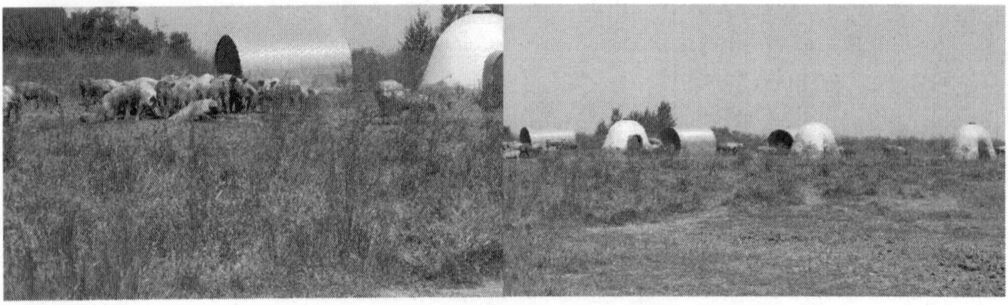

Figure 3.4: Pigs under pasture-based system

3.5 Overview of swine production in India

In India, the swine farming sector is highly unorganized. Pigs are generally reared by economically poor sections of the society, which provide them with better nutritional support and also serves as an important source of livelihood. Pig serves to meet the requirement of the weaker section of the society and also provides a cheap source of healthy animal protein. Around 70% of the pig population is reared under traditional smallholder, low-input demand-driven production system, except for a limited number of semi-commercial pig farms in Kerala, Punjab and Goa. The typical production system consists of a simple pigsty and feeding comprises locally available grains, vegetables and agricultural by-products along with kitchen waste. A total of six pig breeds have been recognized in India. The larger pig population consisting of the non-descript pigs usually have poor production ability and provides a less return to the farmers. Over 20% of the pigs kept in India are crossed with exotic breeds, but with a large proportion of inbreeding because of non-systematic breeding and selection.

Pork production in India is growing at a steady pace. There is stagnancy in the total meat share of pork across the nation. Pig has widely distributed in all the eco-regions of the country and its rearing is an important occupation of the rural society especially amongst the tribal masses. Pigs are concentrated in the north-eastern region where almost 40% of the country's total pig population is reared. According to the latest livestock census (19th Livestock Census, 2012), the pig population of India is 10.29 million and is showing a declining trend. India's pigs constitute about 1% of the world pig population and the piggery sector is gaining slow but steady momentum during the past few years. In the financial year 2014-15 (Government of India), Pork production in India is estimated to be 464 thousand metric tons that contribute nearly 8 percent of the country's animal protein sources. The major pig population of areas are eastern and northeastern regions of the country comprise around 63 percent of the pig population. The highest pig population is in the state of Assam (1.63 million) followed by Uttar Pradesh (1.33 million), Jharkhand (0.96 million), Bihar (0.65 million) and West Bengal (0.65 million). The pork production is concentrated mainly in the states of Uttar Pradesh (30 percent), followed by north-eastern states (25 percent), (Bihar (15 percent), West Bengal (6 percent), Karnataka (4 percent), Jharkhand (4 percent), and Kerala (3 percent).

❑❑❑

Chapter 4

Breeds of Swine

—Dr. Niraj Kumar

The breed can be defined as a group of animals related by descent and similar in most characters like general appearance, features, size, configuration, etc. There may be considerable differences between individuals, still, they have as a group many common points that distinguish them from other groups. Such a common characteristic group is termed a breed. The purity of the breed is maintained by confining the mating of animals within the breed. As per the Animal genetic resources, a total of about 65 different breeds are recognized internationally and the number is expected to increase with the characterization and recognition of breeds by different countries. Breeds of swine can be grouped into two different categories, maternal and terminal breeds. The maternal breeds are known for their large litters and are selected for replacement females. Terminal sire breeds are recognized for their growth and carcass quality and are usually used for terminal crosses. Chester White, Landrace and Yorkshire are the most common maternal breed while Berkshire, Duroc, Hampshire, Spot, Poland China, Pietrain are some of the important terminal sire breeds. The region-wise distribution of major breeds of pig is described as follows:

Indigenous breeds of India: Ghoongroo, Niang Megha, Agonda Goan, Tenyi Vo, Nicobari, Doom, Zovawk and Kaunayen.

Breeds of China: Beijing Black, Fengjing, Meishan, Jiaxing Black, Erhualian and Wuzhishan

Other Asian breeds: Vietnamese Pot-bellied, Cantonese, Malayan, Balinese,Akasai Black Pied, Ba Xuyen and Bangur,

Breeds of Europe: Angeln Saddleback, Basque, Bazna, Belgian Landrace, Bentheim Black Pied, Bulgarian White, Celtic, Chato Murciano, Danish Landrace, Gascon and Juliana,

Many famous breeds of pig are present in the United Kingdom. Some of them are used world-wide for crossbreeding programs.

Breeds of United Kingdom: Berkshire, British Landrace, British Lop, British Saddleback, Cumberland, Essex, Gloucestershire Old Spot, Grice, Hampshire, Large Black, Large White, Middle White, Oxford sandy and black, Small black, Small white, Tamworth, Welsh, Wessex Saddleback and Yorkshire blue and white.

Breeds of United States: American Yorkshire, Chester White, Choctaw, Duroc, Guinea hog, Hereford, Poland China, Red Wattle

4.1 Indigenous Breeds of India

Agonda Goan

Agonda Goan is a local pig breed of the state traditionally known as 'Gavthi Dukor' (village pig). This breed is known for its adaptability and ability to thrive well with available feed resources. It is a small-sized local pig of Goa (India). The body is small to medium-sized, however, the animals maintained on farms are much bigger than the animals in the field. These pigs are mostly black colored with some white patches on legs and face (Figure 4.1). It has rough bristles black and gray in colour. The body weight of an adult male is about 50-60 kg while for an adult female is 30 -100 kg, but may weigh up to 160 kg under good feeding management. The average number of teat is 6 pairs. This breed of a pig plays a major role in the profitability of pig rearing due to faster growth rate, sustainability on scavenging, early maturing and good mothering ability. They are adapted to a hot and humid climate with higher disease resistance and adaptability to stress. People prefer these animals for sausage making. These pigs are difficult to handle as wild in nature. This breed is better for crossbreeding with the exotic breed so as to get better adaptability and disease resistance. Meat is lean with low-fat content with a high dressing percentage (70 - 72%).

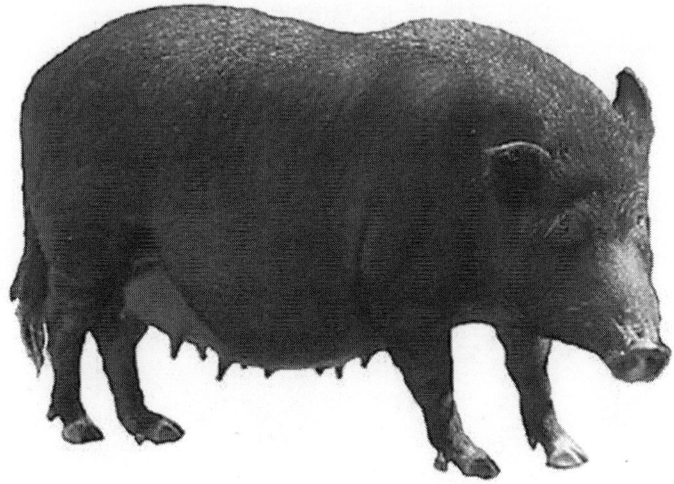

Figure 4.1: Agonda Goan saw.

Tenyi Vo

The new pig breed 'Tenyi Vo' is recorded as a local breed and is indigenous to the districts of Kohima, Peren and Phek of Nagaland State and Senapati district in the Manipur state of India. The nomenclature of the newly recognized breed was also derived since the breed is reared only by the Tenyimi tribes. The breed is considered as the meat of 'very good quality' with a distinctive flavor. The breed is unique for its 'very early sexual maturity' among the male pigs (60-90 days), excellent mothering quality and pendulous belly almost reaching the ground. The pigs have strong and long tapering snout, small erect ears and bright alert eyes. It is predominantly black in colour with white markings on the forehead, flanks and legs (Figure 4.2). The long tail usually ends with a white switch. Adult pig weighs from 35-50 kg and even to the extent of 60-70 kg. It has a life span of 5-6 years. Estimated population is about 60,000-70,000.

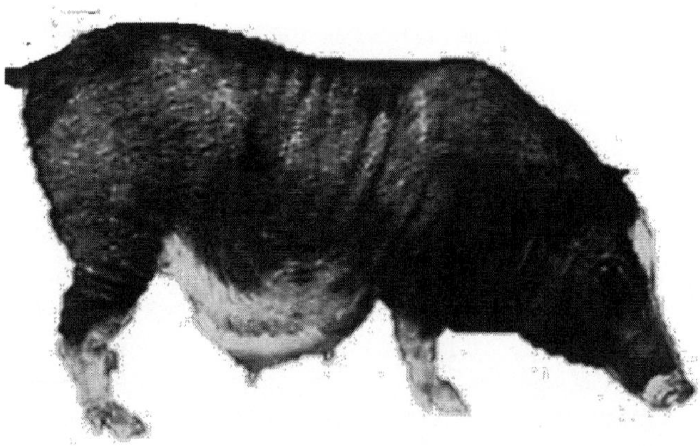

Figure 4.2: Tenyi Vo saw.

Ghoongroo

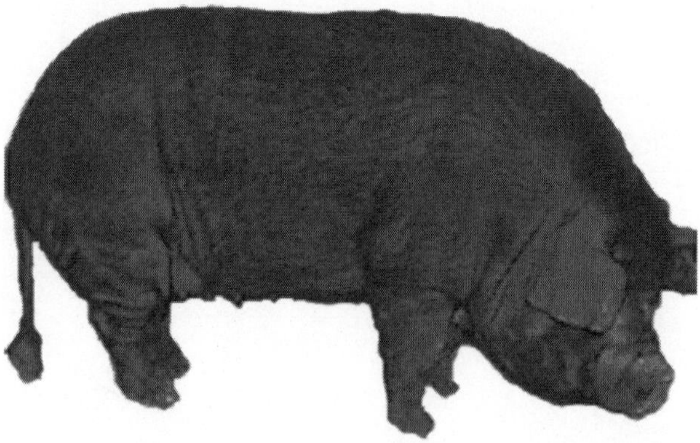

Figure 4.3: Ghoongroo breed.

Ghungroo an indigenous breed of pig from the Tarai region of northeast India particularly north Bengal is popular among the local people because of high prolificacy and ability to sustain in the low input system. This breed produces high-quality pork utilizing agricultural byproducts and kitchen wastes. They are mostly black to tan colour with a broad, flattened face and short, upwardly curved snout gives typical 'Bulldog' facial appearance. Ears resembling those of the elephant's ears and are pendulous, large and heart-shaped that are very distinct for identification. The body top line is straight with a flat type belly (Figure 4.3). Bristles are thick, coarse and long. The sows bear 5- 6 pairs of teats with the ability to give birth of average 9-10 piglets per farrowing. The average birth weights of the piglets are around 700g respectively. At 3 months of age, the average body weights of male and female piglets were 11.5 and 11 kg respectively. Both sexes are very much docile and easy to handle. Sows show an excellent mothering ability which is an important trait in relation to piglet survivability. At the National Research Centre on Pig, Rani, Guwahati, Ghungroo pigs are being maintained under an intensive system of rearing with standard breeding, feeding and management system. The performance of this indigenous pig is good in terms of productive and reproductive efficiency.

Niang Megha

Niang Megha is a medium sized pig breed from Garo, Khasi and Jaintia hills of Meghalaya reared mainly for pork and bristle. The animals have typical wild look with erect bristles on dorsal midline. The coat colour of Niang Megha population was observed to be of two types i.e. solid black and black with white patches on forehead and legs (Figure 4.4). Ears are small and erect which is extended vertically. The shape of the head is long and straight. The number of teats ranged between 5 and 6 pairs. The age at first mating is over 8 months. The breed farrow first time between 11-12 months and farrowing interval is around 7 months. Average litter size is around 6.

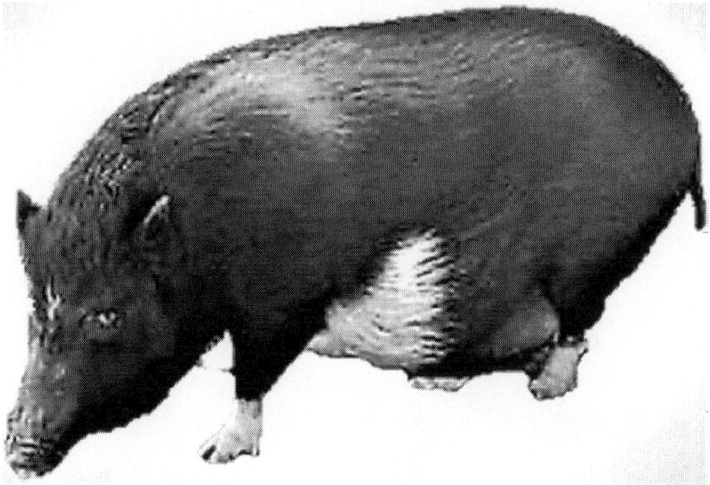

Figure 4.4: Niang Megha breed.

Nicobari

The Nicobari pig, locally known as 'Ha-un' is indigenous pig germplasm located only in the Nicobar group of islands of India and is reared by Nicoabri tribes with an estimated population of about 35,000. They are a fast runners. This breed plays a significant role in the Nicobari community's tradition and culture. The majority of the pigs appear short with a long body, and their skin color includes black, gray, brown, and blackish brown (Figure 4.5). The adult body varies from 26 to 61kg. The average age at first farrowing is around 11 months with a farrowing interval of about 7 months. The average number of litter size is 7. The number of teats ranged from five to six pairs indicating higher fecundity. This indigenous pig breed is healthy, active, and well adapted to the local environment of Nicobar. They can survive with a very low level of management. Currently, the breed is under the endangered category. The low-input pig production system in the present study both is sustainable and is in accordance with the tribal farmers' traditional practice. The pigs are having good mothering characteristics.

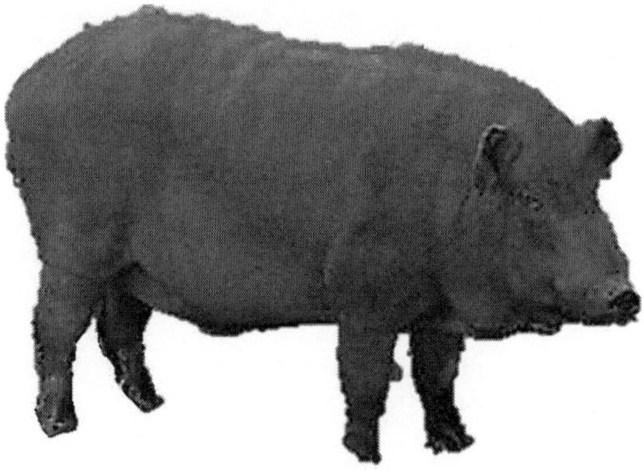

Figure 4.5: Nicobari pig

Doom

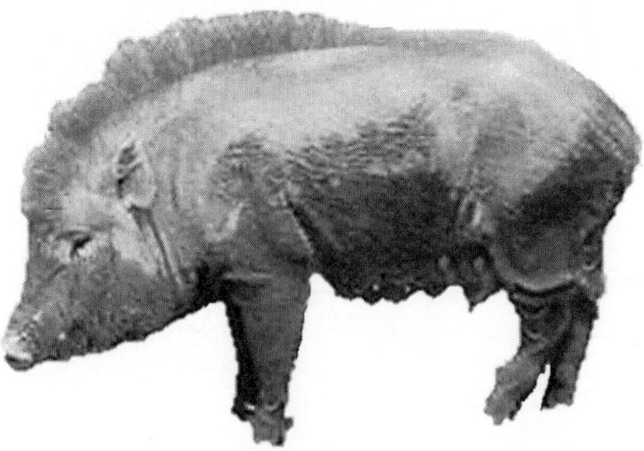

Figure 4.6: Doom pig

The distribution of Doom pigs are in Bongaigaon, Kokrajhar and Dhubri districts of Assam state. The estimated population is about 3,000. These are medium-sized animal with black in colour and have a short concave and pointed snout. Hard and long bristles (erected mane) are spreading from forehead to back of the shoulder (Figure 4.6). The shape of the head is long and straight. The ear is short, erect and pointed upward. The adult body varies from 36 to 50kg. The number of teats ranged between 5 and 6 pairs. The average litter size is around 5 with the birth weight of piglet around 700g. The average body weight at 7-8 months is around 35kg.

Zovawk

Zovawk pig is present in a different parts of Mizoram state in India. The population size is small and outnumbered by the crossbreed population. They are of small size and attain puberty at the age of 2.5 months when they are about 4.5 kg body weight. The first farrowing occurs at the age of 9-10 months when they are of about 40 kg body weights. Their coat colour is black with a white patch on the legs. They are short-legged with small and erect ears, the face is narrow and long tapering towards the snout which is moderately curved (Figure: 4.7). The average litter size at birth is 6. The average birth weight of piglets is around 500gm. In Mizoram, the pig is one of the most valued and popular as 100% tribal population in the region are pork eaters. The Zovawk pork is preferred by the people of Mizoram due to its taste and perceived medicinal properties as conceived by local people. This pig is of scavenging type and very popular amongst the pig farmers in the state for its ability to sustain in a low input system. The pig is very alert to the social happening such as the presence of an intruder in the farm by making an immediate response to the sound or the gestures of the intruder.

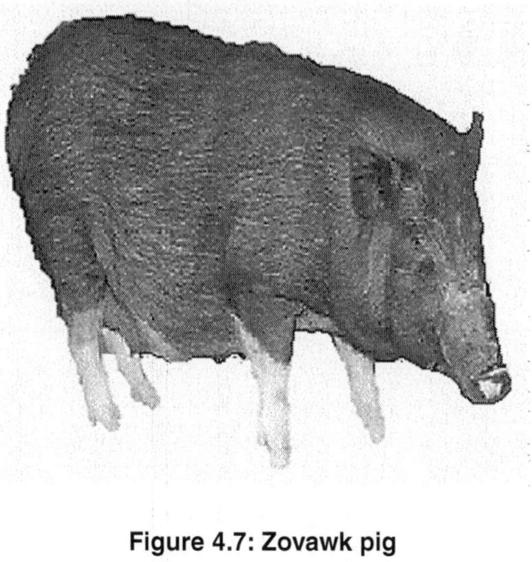

Figure 4.7: Zovawk pig

4.2 Breed of Pig from China

Breeds of China: Beijing Black, Fengjing, Meishan, Jiaxing black, Erhualian and Wuzhishan

Beijing Black (Peking Black)

The Beijing Black is a domestic pig from China mainly black in color, but has some white markings. The breed is developed by crossbreeding a Berkshire with a common Chinese pig.

Fengjing pig

Fengjing is a large black pig. It has large floppy ears. It has a highly wrinkled face and wrinkled body. This breed has very high rates of breeding, producing two litters per year. The average litter size is around 17-20. The pig grows at a slower rate and has a good, juicy taste. Western countries are using this pig in the female line of a breeding program for improving the taste, disease resistance and litter size.

Meishan

Meishan is slow-growing pig. It is a black colored breed with short legs, big stomach, deep back, large drooping ears and wrinkled black skin.

This breed is best known for its high prolificacy with a litter size of 14 -17 with an average birth weight 900gm, with weaning of 11 – 12. They are having 8-9 pairs of teats. Daily weight gain is 300 – 400 gm with feed conversion ratio (FCR) 5:1. An adult male weight about 450 kg and a female weight 350 kg average. Due to its fecundity, it was imported to the United States in the late 1980s. It has an early age of maturity with an abundance of fat.

Wuzhishan

It is a miniature pig and is a new medical and life science experimental model animal.

4.3 Major Breeds of Swine Across the World

Berkshire

Berkshire is originated in Berkshire County, England and is one of the oldest improved breeds of swine. The first Berkshires were brought to the U.S. in 1823. Like all the swine breeds that end in the shire, Berkshires have erect ears. In fact, the word shire means erect. The Berkshire breed has a color pattern consisting of only white and black hairs. While the original Berkshire pig was sandy-brown, modern Berkshire pigs are almost entirely black, with six white points composed of four white feet, some white on the face, and a white switch on the tail. More than 10% of the body in white markings is a disqualification for registration of this breed. They are a short-legged breed. The most distinctive characteristic of Berkshire is its head. The snout is short and turned up, and the ears are erect (Figure 4.8).

The Berkshire breed has excellent efficiency in gaining weight. It is an early maturing breed and producing plenty of lean meat even on small joints. The meat of Berkshire is praised for a greater proportion of lean meat intermixed with streaks of fat. This intramuscular fat gives more marbling in comparison to other breeds. After cooking, the pork is having a juicy flavor due to increased marbling. The average weight at maturity is around 600 pounds (270 kg). Being an excellent mother and good forager, Berkshire is ideal for the smallholder. It is hardy, docile, economical and early maturing, and is often referred to by the Japanese as being 'the best pork in the world' (known in Japan as Kurobuta Pork).

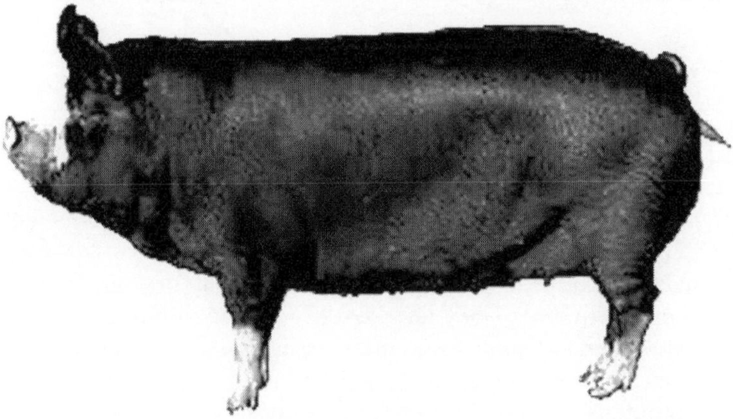

Figure 4.8: Berkshire breed

Chester White

The Chester White breed was developed in Chester and Delaware Counties in Pennsylvania, the USA from parent stock of Cheshire, Lincolnshire, and Yorkshire breeding, all of which were of English origin. These are large-sized breed with solid white in color and small, downward-pointing ears (Figure 4.9).

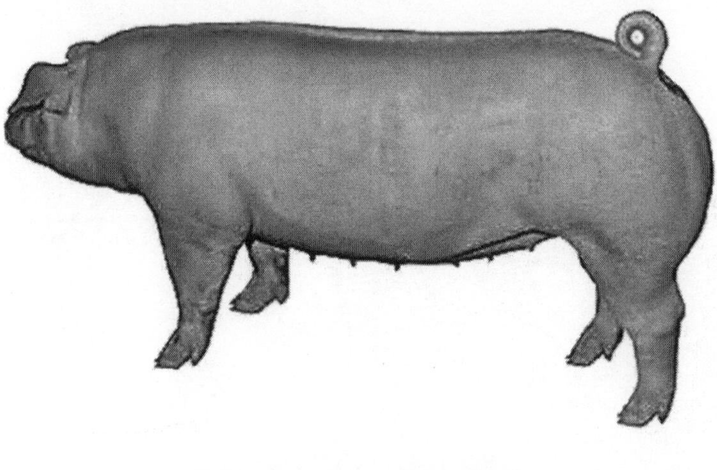

Figure 4.9: Chester White breed

Sows of this breed are noted for their prolificacy and mothering ability because they produce large litters of pigs that grow out rapidly. This breed is versatile and suitable for both intensive and extensive husbandry. Sows and boars are used for producing hybrids meat hogs. Among white breeds of pig, the Chester White is the most durable as it can gain as much as 1.36 pounds (0.62 kg) a day. For the production of 1 pound (0.45 kg) of pork, 3 pounds (1.4 kg) of grain is required. The Chester Whites are prone to sunburn due to pale body color hence shade is required during summer. Meat is lean and well-marbled with good flavor.

Duroc

The breed was developed in the United States and is a choice for many mixed-breed commercial hogs. The breed is red colored with shades varying from a cherry red to golden colour. A thick auburn winter coat and hard skin allow them to survive the cold. The molting of coat occurs in summer and pig appear almost bald, but as a consequence, it can cope with hot dry summers equally well. The ears are drooping and not held erect, covering the eyes (Figure 4.10). It is a robust and heavy-boned breed. Duroc pig is well-known to have an excellent weight gain rate and as a high feed converter. They have large-framed, medium length, and muscular bodies with good carcass quality and body weights of about 400 kg and 350 kg for mature boar and mature sow respectively. The sow matures early, produces large litter up to 15 piglets and good mothering ability. They have excellent feed intake to produce large quantities of milk. They are having an excellent reputation for performances well in tough conditions. Due to good disease resistance ability, they are fit for outdoor and extensive pig keeping systems. Durocs have been identified as a superior genetics source for improving quality. Their muscle quality and their ability to grow fast have made them an outstanding terminal sire. This is one of the most popular breeds because of distinguished accomplishments in longevity and prolificness in the female line and lean gain efficiency, carcass yield, and product quality in the terminal sire.

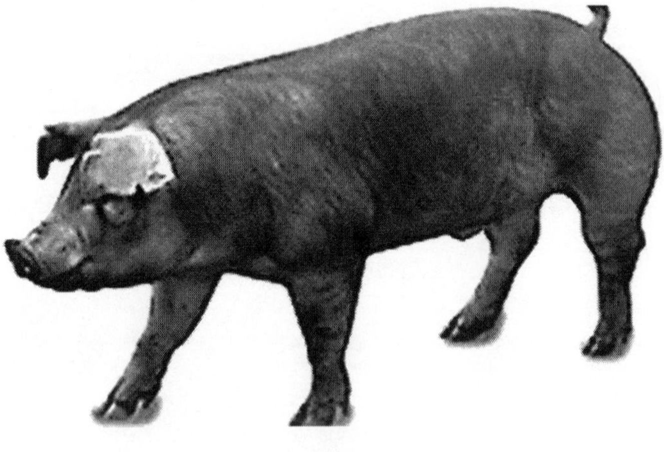

Figure 4.10: Duroc breed

Gloucestershire Old Spot

This breed originated in the Berkeley Valley region of England. Now it spread throughout the United Kingdom. It is the oldest spotted pedigree pig breed in the world. It is named after the county of Gloucestershire. The Gloucestershire Old

Spots is predominantly white in colour with black spots. Selection of this breed is done with less black and now only a spot or two are usually found. Head is of long length with a slightly dished nose. The ears are well set apart, dropping forward to the nose which almost covers the face of a mature pig and hangs towards the nose (Figure 4.11). Legs are straight and strong. They are among the large size pigs in England. They are known for docility, intelligence, and prolificacy. The mature weight of the boar is 600 lb (272 kg) and sows 500 lb (227 kg). The breed is good foragers and the sows are having good maternal skills to raise large litters of piglets on pasture. The sows produce large litters and a high amount of milk.

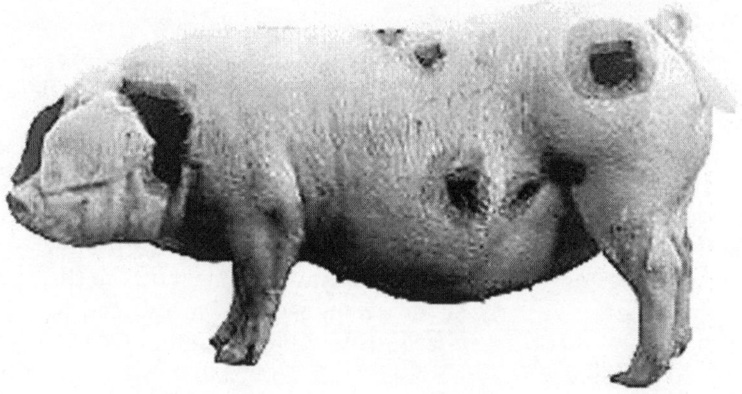

Figure 4.11: Gloucestershire Old Spots breed

Hampshire

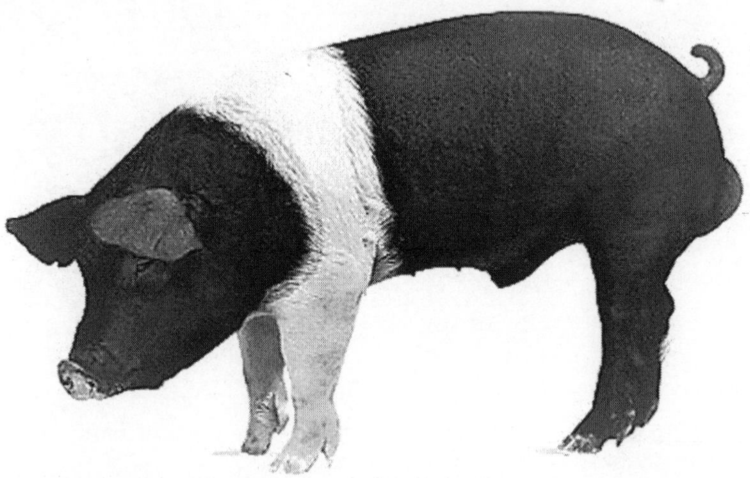

Figure 4.12: Hampshire breed

The Hampshire breed originated in southern Scotland and Northern England. They are black in colour with a white band around the body at the shoulder including the front legs and feet. The head, tail and back legs are black (Figure 4.12). Their ears are erect and their face is longer and straighter than other breeds. They are known for being heavy muscled, lean, aggressive hogs with large loin eye areas, and possess less back fat. They have thin skin, which makes processing easier. Hence, Hampshire boars are considered good terminal sires. Hampshire sows are good tampered, very prolific, have extra longevity and are good mothers. They have been used extensively in crossbreeding because of their good carcass quality. The growth is not as fast as many crossbreds, but they do grow faster than Yorkshires.

Yorkshire

The Yorkshire is also known as the Large White breed. The breed was developed in the County of York in England. The Yorkshire was imported to the USA around 1830 from England to Ohio. Today they are one of the most recorded breeds of swine in the United States. Yorkshires are entirely white, with ears that are erect and moderate in size. They possess moderately long head, have a slightly dished face and a broad snout (Figure 4.13). The neck is long, fine and evenly full to shoulders with deep and wide chests and they have level, long and wide back. An adult male weights around 300 to 400 kg and an adult sow weighs around 230 to 320 kg. Yorkshires are recognized worldwide as the mother breed due to their prolificacy and mothering ability. The Large White is a rugged and hardy breed and withstands variations in climate and other environmental factors. For these reasons, it has been used widely in crossbreeding programs. Their ability to improve other breeds by crossing has truly made them a breed of choice in commercial swine are produced. The breed is known for its high-quality bacon and pork are sought.

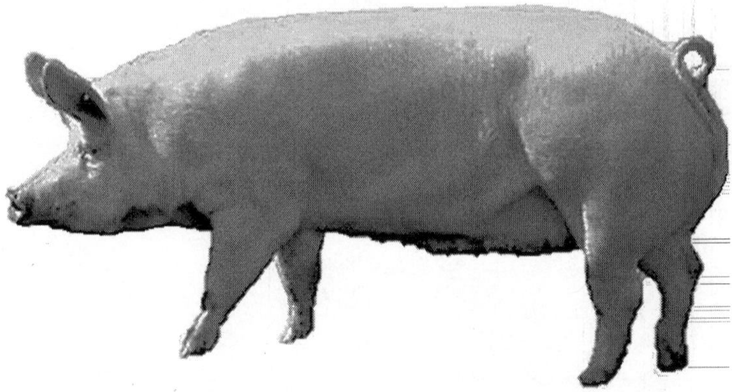

Figure 4.13: Yorkshire breed

Landrace

The breed originated in Europe. The breed has white skin and hair while small black spots on the skin are common. They have a long, deep side, a flatter back, a straight snout and a trim jowl. The long, drooping ears cover a portion of the face (Figure 4.14). Landrace sows are prolific, possess good mothering ability, farrow large litters and good milking ability. The breed is medium in size. They are excellent for efficient feed utilization with meaty carcass and have a high dressing percentage. Landrace is known for their mothering ability and prolificacy but are also selected for leanness and muscle in many countries of the world. Landrace breeds are well-known breed for their ability to cross with other breeds. They are also known for their length of the body. Many breed strains exist within the Landrace population, including American Landrace, Belgian Landrace, Dutch Landrace, Finnish Landrace, French Landrace, German Landrace, Italian Landrace, British Landrace and Swedish Landrace. The American Landrace came from descendants of the Danish Landrace that had its origin in 1895.

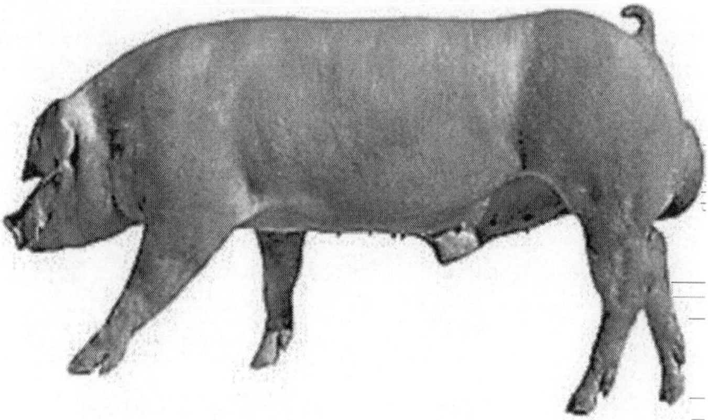

Figure 4.14: Landrace breed

Poland China

Poland China was developed in the Miami Valley region of Warren and Butler Counties in Ohio. Parent stock used in developing the breed was the Big China Hog from Pennsylvania, the Irish Grazer from Ireland, the White Byfield Hog from Russia, the Berkshire, and native hogs. In color, Poland China is black with six white points (Figure 4.15).

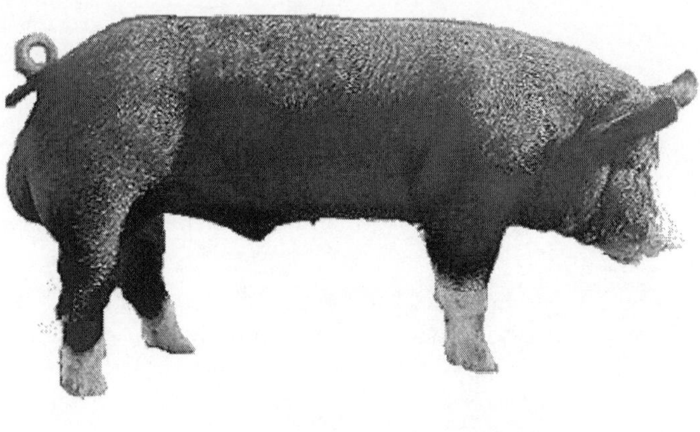

Figure 4.15: Poland China breed

These points include a blazing white face, white feet, and a white tip on the tail. Poland Chinas are a large breed. Ears are droopy and head appear well trimmed are characteristic of these hogs. It has strong bone and well-developed legs and feet. It is prolific (produce 16 – 17 piglets per farrow) and good meat and carcass quality. It is also a good converter of feed to meat and attains maturity early. A mature boar weighs between 250 kg and 360 kg and a mature sow weighs between 225 kg and 300 kg. The typical Poland China has thick hams with good length and produces highly desirable carcasses.

Tamworth

The Tamworth is a breed of domestic pig originating in Tamworth, United Kingdom, with input from Irish pigs and are known for being a bacon type hog. This breed exhibits an elongated head shape, long neck and legs, deep sides but narrow backs. The ears are erect and pointed (Figure 4.16). The breed is having a good skeletal system and excellent foot structure. Colors range from a pale gingery to dark mahogany red with straight hair. Tamworths are a medium-sized swine breed. The adult boar ranging from 250 to 370 kg (550 to 820 lb) and the mature sow from 200 to 300 kg (440 to 660 lb). Litter sizes are typically somewhat smaller than commercial breeds.

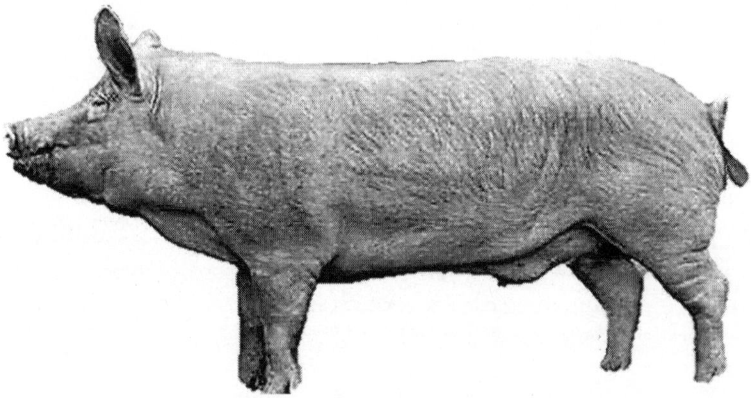

Figure 4.16: Tamworth breed

Pietrain

Originated in the village of Pietrain, Belgium. The breed is of medium size and is white with black spots (Figure 4.17). The black spots are encircled by characteristic rings of light pigmentation that carries white hair. The black hair is not as deeply pigmented.

The ears of the breed are erect and commonly referred to as being of piebald markings. Pietrains have been selected for extremely lean carcasses with a large volume of muscle. The Pietrain breed is very popular in its native country. It was exported to other countries, especially Germany. They are used primarily as a terminal sire breed throughout Europe

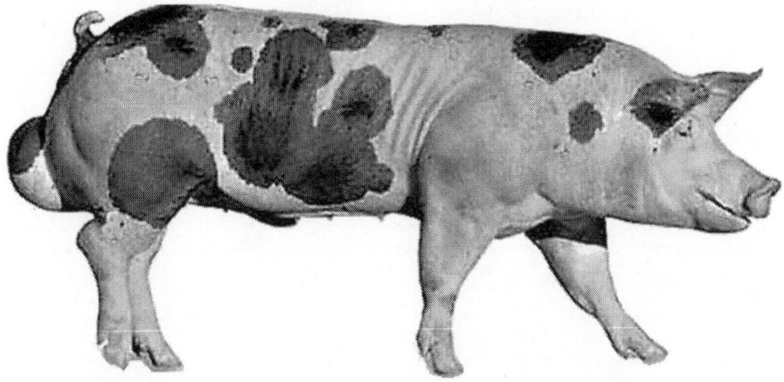

Figure 4.17: Pietrain breed

Vietnamese Potbelly

A dwarf swine breed of Vietnam with an average weight of approximately 50 kg. It is uniformly black, with heavily wrinkled skin. It has a large sagging belly, which sows may drag on the ground in pregnant. The head is small, with an up-turned snout, small ears and eyes, and heavy sagging jowls (Figure 4.18). Being a small pig, they produce select cuts of meat and a lot of sausage and bacon.

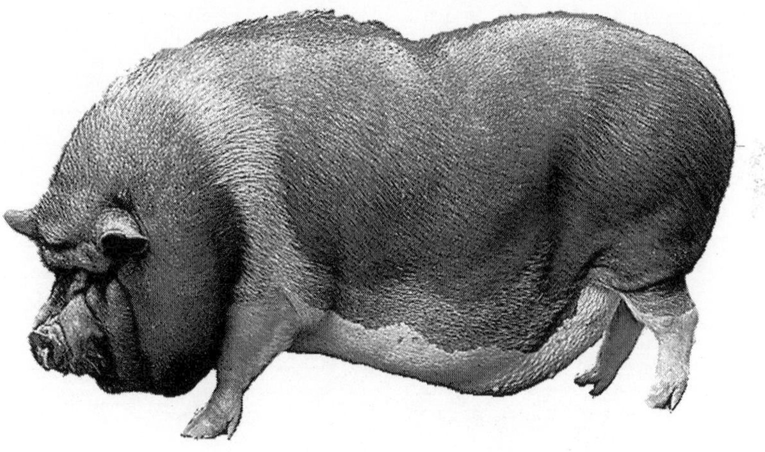

Figure 4.18: Vietnamese Potbelly breed

❑❑❑

Chapter 5

Management of Basic Swine Activities

—Dr. Niraj Kumar & Dr. Yohannes Tekle

5.1 Collection of Blood Sample

A blood sample is collected from the pig for many purposes like to know the health status and blood parameters of the pig. It is also collected for conducting research activities. Restraining is done as per age and behavior of the pig. Restraint such as snout tying and squeeze chutes should be avoided in research studies conducted on swine. These methodologies are stressful to the pig and make it more difficult for personnel to interact with the animals when they are on a chronic study. Vocalization during this type of restraint is also stressful for personnel who are working with the animals. The stress response also causes variability in many blood values. Swine may be restrained in humane restraint slings or with the use of minimal manual restrain in smaller animals. Chemical restraining may be used for large pigs during research activities. Syringes, needles and vacutainers of various capacities are required as per the size of animals and the site of a collection of blood. Surgical spirit, cotton wool, labels, rope, ear muffs and two handlers are also required.

Collection of Blood from Ear Vein

The ear veins are located along the cranial and caudal edges of the ear. The veins are raised by applying digital pressure of the ear. The skin is cleaned with cotton wool and surgical spirit. The artery is present as a central vessel on the ear. A 20-22 g, 1″ needles can be used depending on the thickness of the veins of the pig. Store blood in a glass vacutainer tube. Only 1-2 ml of blood can usually be obtained from the ear vein. A catheter can be used to collect blood from ear vain which can be maintained successfully for up to 3 days and blood can be drained any amount as per requirement.

Collection of Blood from Anterior Vena Cava

From this site, blood can be collected from all sizes of pigs. The cranial vena cava (precava) is the largest vessel that is commonly accessed for blood samples. Animals may be positioned in a restraint sling or placed in dorsal recumbency to access this vessel. The vessel is always accessed from the right side of the thoracic inlet to avoid the vagus and recurrent laryngeal nerves which are more prominent on the left side. The skin is cleaned with cotton wool and surgical spirit. The needle is advanced at a 450 angle towards the left shoulder of the pig. Repeated blood sampling from this area will result in hematoma or blood clot formation in the thoracic inlet because it is not possible to stop leakage from the venipuncture with digital pressure. In swine less than 50 kg body weight, the vessel can be accessed using a 20 g, 1.5″ needle. For animals more than 50 kg body weight, needles as large as 18 g, 2.5″ may have to be used.

Collection of Blood from a Cephalic Vein

The cephalic vein can be accessed along the cranial surface of the radius on the foreleg and also as it crosses the ventral surface of the neck to enter the external jugular vein at the thoracic inlet. A tourniquet is placed around the foreleg at the level of the proximal radius and the elbow (ulnar head) is pressed to extend the leg. In order to access the vessel on the ventral surface of the neck the animal is placed in dorsal recumbency and digital pressure is applied to the thoracic inlet alongside the trachea. The skin is cleaned with cotton wool and surgical spirit. The cephalic vein can then be visualized. This vessel can be accessed with a 20 g, 1.0″ needle. The amount of blood that can be withdrawn is usually less than 5 ml.

Collection of blood from femoral vein and artery

The femoral artery and vein are located in the femoral groove formed by the borders of the sartorius and gracilis muscles. They may be appreciated by palpation of the pulse or by following the pulse of the medial saphenous artery which vanishes as this superficial vessel enters into the femoral groove. The vessels are located under the medial edge of the gracilis muscle rather than directly in the groove. The pig is positioned in dorsal recumbency and gentle extension of the rear leg will provide access to this site. The skin is cleaned with cotton wool and surgical spirit. Sedation is required for this procedure. The femoral vessels can be accessed with 20 g, 1.0-1.5″ needles. The amount of blood that can be withdrawn is usually 5-10 ml.

Collection of blood from a cranial abdominal (external mammary) vein

The cranial abdominal vein is located along the deep lateral edge of the first three mammary glands. This vessel greatly enlarges in farrowed sows. To distend this vessel digital pressure is applied at the caudal edge of the last rib along the line of mammary glands. The skin is cleaned with cotton wool and surgical spirit. The needle of 20 g, 1.0″ can be used for blood collection. Only 5 ml of blood can be obtained in pigs which have not reached sexual maturity. In already farrowed sows 20 ml of blood volume can be obtained.

Tail (Coccygeal) Vein

Blood can be collected from this site at any size of the pig but the amount of blood to be collected is usually less i.e. 0.5ml in piglets up to 2 ml in adult pigs. The coccygeal veins accompany the artery on the ventral surface of the tail. These vessels may be accessed by raising the tail and performing venipuncture at the base of the tail. The needle of 20 g, 1.0″ can be used for blood collection. Only 1-2 ml of blood can be obtained from these vessels.

Collection of blood from a jugular vein

This method of blood collection is used to collect blood from 30kg pig to adult. Restraining of the pig is needed. The internal jugular vein, carotid artery and vagus nerve are all located in a sheath on either side of the trachea on the ventral surface of the cervical vertebrae. The positioning of the head and neck are the same as for the external jugular vein. The carotid pulse can be used to locate these vessels. The vein will be slightly lateral to the artery and the nerve and nearly 25 to 40 mm below the skin generally. The carotid artery is frequently used as the vascular access site for terminal bleeding under general anesthesia. These vessels can be accessed with a 20 g, 1.0-1.5″ needle. Bradycardia or arrhythmias may occur if the vagus nerve is accidentally stimulated with the needle. (Figure 3)

5.2 Intubation of Stomach Tube

This process is required for feeding orphan piglets with colostrum. Piglets may need supplemental colostrum or milk if they are not strong enough to suckle, or if they are unable to gain sufficient access to a sow (e.g. through the death of the sow or insufficient teats). If a piglet is having a suckling reflex bottle feeding of colostrum or milk can be done. If there is no sucking reflex, then the administration of the fluid using a stomach tube should be done. Dextrose sugar solution can also be given to provide an instant source of energy. A plastic stomach tube of 4mm diameter is used for intubation and a syringe of the required capacity for introducing colostrum or dextrose is needed. Before the inserting tube it is lubricated either with colostrum or liquid paraffin. The syringe is also filled with a desirable solution to be injected. Then piglets are held under the arm with a hand over the head then stimulated for suckling reflex by placing a little finger at the back of the tongue. The third finger is then placed in the angle of the jaw. Then lubricated is inserted over the back of the tongue and gently pushed in the feeling for a swallowing reflex. Piglet will cough violently if the tube is inserted accidentally into the trachea. In such condition, tube is removed and tried again. A resistance will be felt after the tube enters the stomach. Usually, 10-30 ml solution is inserted at one time. Insertion of more liquid may lead to vomition. This process may be repeated every two hours if needed.

5.3 Body Condition Scoring of Pig

Body Condition Scoring can contribute significantly to the good management of sows in all settings. Body condition scoring provides a clear indication of both the appropriateness of the feed and the effectiveness of the feed delivery system. The expectation of consistent high performance puts a heavy burden on the energy reserves of lean genotype sows. It is therefore very important that they build up fat cover before their first service in order to maintain good conditions throughout their productive life.Condition scoring aims to give guidelines to achieve adequate nutrition that minimizes the risk of welfare problems in the sow. Condition scoring is a hands-on technique. It is not sufficient just to examine the sow by eye, it is essential to feel the amount of fat she has covering her bones. The main areas to feel are the hips bones and along the backbone.It can also be useful to feel the two pointed bones either side of the tail, the "pin bones", and observe how much of a cavity there is, if any, under the base of the tail. The best way to feel is with the palm of the hand rather than with the fingers.The body condition of sows is scored from 1 (emaciated) to 5 (obese) (figure 5.1). The ideal body condition of a sow at farrowing is 3 and at weaning about 2. Young sows (first and second parity) in very poor condition at weaning may be better mated on the second heat. Trials have shown that skipping a heat can improve litter size.

Condition score 1 (Emaciated)

The backbone is very prominent and can be felt with little pressure. This animal's skeletal structure can be easily seen and palpated. The pelvic bone is very prominent and there is a deep cavity around the tail head. Due to a lack of fat cover, the ribs and backbone are easily differentiated. The loin muscle is very shallow with a hollow flank. The ribs and bone structures are visible with no fat cover and are very prominent. There is no fat between muscle and skin.

Condition score 2 (Thin)

The spinous processes are still extended, but less sharp, and can be felt with pressure. The loin area is narrow and the flank is hollow. There is a slight cover on the spine but the vertebrae are prominent. The rib cage is less apparent but individual ribs can easily be detected with slight pressure.

Condition score 3 (Ideal)

This animal has a good muscle to fat ratio. The optimum amount of fat cover over the shoulders, loin, ribs and tail head. Hips and spinous processes are not visible and smooth to touch but can be palpated with pressure. The loin muscle is filled with a cover of fat. there is a more rounded top due to increased fill in the loin. Sows should not enter the farrowing house with a condition of less than 3.

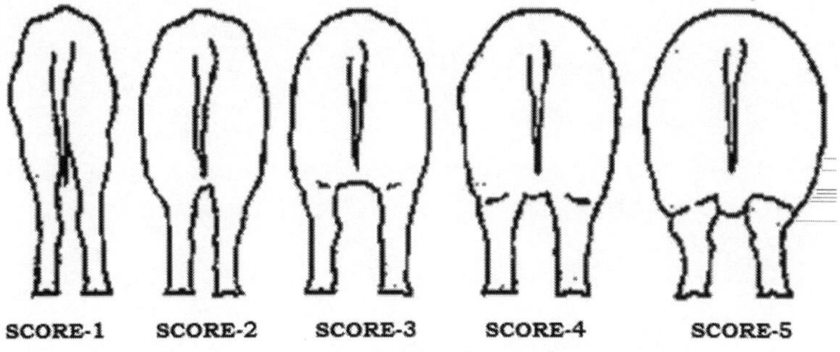

Figure 5.1: Body condition score of the pig.

Condition score 4 (Fat)

The entire animal appears smooth and has an enlarged, rounded appearance. Pelvic bones can only be felt with firm pressure. There is no cavity around the tail. The flank area is filled. By applying firm pressure, the edge of transverse spinal processes can be felt. Vertebrae can felt only with firm pressure. The rib cage is not visible and it is difficult to feel ribs. There is more fat cover over the shoulder, loins, and ribs.

Condition score 5 (Obase)

The animal is more rounded than an animal with a lower-body condition score (because of fat deposits). Bone and muscle definition can not be seen. The animal's top appears flat because of increased fat in the loin and pelvic area. There is no visible bone structure. The spine cannot be felt. Due to fat deposition around the shoulder, the neck appears shorter. The hip, loin, and tail head have a flat look as engulfed in heavy fat cover.

❑❑❑

Chapter 6

Housing of Pig

—Mr. Tsegay Tkue

6.1 Site Selection for Swine Farming

Careful selection of the site before establishing a swine farm is important to prevent management, welfare and environmental problems. There are several factors which determine the best site for swine facilities are described below.

Space

Adequate space should be available so that farm can be expanded in the future. Space for vehicle access and area for parking should be considered. It should be away from the city or human population. Such a community should be avoided that has religious taboo for pigs.

Topography and drainage

Factors that make sites unsuitable are high rainfall, poor drainage and stony (flinty) soils. A dry lying area is essential for the comfort of all pigs. Wet paddocks allow water and mud to be trampled into the huts. Wet muddy areas lead to feed being trampled and wasted and feed levels may have to be increased for pigs to get their appropriate ration. Waterlogging can also make it difficult for pigs to get to the feeding areas, water troughs and huts. Stony soils and thin soils over rock, especially those containing flints, can damage legs and feet which become infected. Waterlogged soils can lead to a softening of feet making injury and infection more likely.Piglets are particularly susceptible to chilling and hypothermia from wet bedding which increases their risk susceptibility to disease.

Sun and wind

The risk of chilling, particularly of piglets, is significantly increased when temperatures are low and wind-chill factors are high. The effects of wind-chill can be reduced by the selection of sites that offer natural shelter either from the surrounding topography or natural windbreaks such as hedges. The long axis of the farm should be in a north-south direction so that the orientation should be in the east-west direction to allow sunlight to enter in the morning and evening. The building should be constructed in such a way that direct sunlight can reach the platforms, gutters and mangers. Protection from sunlight during hot weather particularly in tropics should be considered. The roof should be made of a material that protects the pig from rain and direct sunlight.

Availability of Water

A year-round supply of potable water is essential to any pig unit. Remote sites can present difficult problems in achieving an adequate supply of water for the stock.

Accessibility

Easy accessibility is required for the transfer of stock while purchasing or sale. Close access to the market will reduce transportation cost. The farm should be connected with a broad road.

Electricity

Light is required for many farm operations. Hence, it is necessary to have an uninterrupted electricity supply on the farm.

Labor

Honest, economic and regular supply of labor is required for profitable swine farming.

Security

Security against theft and fire is necessary. Limiting farm visitors access to control disease and to reduce interference with farm work is also necessary.

6.2 Pig housing

The efficiency of intensive housing units of the pig is strongly influenced by temperature control and ventilation. The space and the length of feeding troughs and the comfort and facilities of pens play an important role in optimum pig production. Intensive pig housing requires planning for economical building construction to produce the maximum amount of quality meat in the shortest possible time.Pigs at different stages of growth have different environmental and climatic requirements. In order to reach their full potential, boars and sows especially need special attention as far as prevention of high ambient temperatures and other stress factors are concerned.

6.2.1 Ventilation control in intensive pig production units

Ventilation means the exchange of air inside a farm building with fresh outside air. The objective of ventilation is the control of the ambient temperature and humidity, the provision of fresh air, the removal of harmful gases and the movement of air. The level of air circulation, dust levels, relative humidity, temperature and gas concentrations must be kept within the prescribed limit so that it will not be harmful to the animals. Efficient ventilation systems is required in commercial (intensive) pig production facilities to maintain the temperature, moisture and air pollution caused by feed, feces and pig itself under desirable limit. Mechanical ventilation (air and temperature conditioning) is indeed used, especially for piglets that are weaned early at three weeks. However, the installation cost is very high. Buildings with natural ventilation are more economical in terms of fixed and running costs.

Temperature

Controlled ventilation is to control the rate at which the air is replaced. The micro ambient temperature is the temperature around each pig and it can be effectively managed by means of ventilation. Pigs that are herded together in a building create heat. The heat may be applied to good effect during cold conditions, but during warm conditions, it must be removed by means of effective ventilation. The temperature usually increases when the temperature inside the building rises above the outside temperature due to heat emitted by the pigs. Temperatures inside buildings can be controlled effectively with the use of natural ventilation, provided that the design of the building, as well as the layout and construction, are done properly. Effective ventilation is essential to the wellbeing of the stock as it provides fresh air, removes noxious gases and aids in controlling temperature. Excessive heat loss should be prevented either by the structural insulation of the external walls, roof and the floor in the lying area or by the provision of adequate bedding. Heat gain to buildings in hot conditions will be minimized by the insulation in the walls and roof. Pigs are having limited ability to sweat hence they highly susceptible to heat stress. Possible cooling methods, including blowing air over the pigs, providing water spray/misting systems or simply wetting floors with a hosepipe, can be used to ensure that pigs in buildings do not become overheated in hot weather. The provision of some dry lying area must be considered so that pigs can move away from wet and cold conditions. Live weight, group size, floor type, airspeed and feed intake markedly affect temperature requirements and stock-keepers must take these factors into account when determining the minimum temperature appropriate in each case. The temperature requirements increase with low feeding level and slatted floors while the requirement decreases when pig are provided with straw bedding, higher body weight of pigs with high feed level. Abrupt fluctuations in temperature in housing systems within any 24-hour period should be avoided. Wide fluctuations in the daily temperature regime can create stress that may trigger outbreaks of vice, such as tail biting, or disease such as pneumonia. The normal minimum temperature requirement within the range is as per the table 6.1.

Table 6.1: Recommended Thermal Conditions for Swine

Type and weight	*Preferred range*
Lactating sow and litter	60-800F for sow; piglets have 900F creep area
Prenursery (5-15kg)	80 to 900F
Nursery (15-35kg)	65 to 800F
Growing (35-70kg)	60 to 750F
Finishing (70-100kg)	50 to 750F
Sows or boars	60 to 750F

Source: Adapted from NRC (1981)

Humidity

It plays an important part in the microclimate conditions inside piggeries. Try to maintain the relative humidity between 50% and 60% to minimize the growth of disease microorganisms. Some disease microorganisms grow rapidly at a humidity above 60% while others grow well at low humidity. When ventilation is sufficient to keep the humidity below 60% other contaminants, such as gases and respirable dust, tend to be low as well. High relative humidity promotes rapid corrosion of metal equipment, creating an additional expense. High relative humidity also leads to more rapid deterioration of the electrical system.Relative humidity values of more than 80% and less than 40% should be avoided. This may be brought about randomly by means of natural ventilation, or by means of controlled ventilation and proper management.

Major gases

Suggested allowable concentrations of the three common gases ammonia, carbon dioxide and hydrogen sulfide found in swine buildings should not be more than 10, 3000 and 5 ppm, respectively. These concentrations are easily achieved with an adequate ventilation system. Harmful gases should be removed for the sake of the pig's health. The building should be managed in such a way that it requires the minimum amount of air changes to regulate the temperature. At the same time, it has to be ensured that gases, dust particles and pathogens are removed effectively. At higher concentrations, each of these gases can be detrimental to animal and human health and to productivity. Dust is an irritant that can increase respiratory problems in both swine and humans. Adding fats or oils to the feed can remove more than half of the total room dust.

Light and noise

Where pigs are kept in a building, adequate lighting must be available to enable them to be thoroughly inspected at any time. Pigs kept in buildings must be kept with an appropriate period of rest from artificial lighting. Artificial lighting with an intensity of at least 40 lux must be provided for a minimum period of 8 hours per day.Exposuretoconstant (noiselevels above 85dBA)orsuddennoise should be avoided. The siting of machinery such as feed milling units should be appropriate to minimize the noise impact on the housed stock.

Sensors

The use of sensors is to regulate an environmental modification system. They should be placed where they can monitor conditions representative of the microenvironment. They should be maintained and calibrated regularly.

Emergency Precautions

Precautions for some emergency conditions in farms, such as fire, flood, or disruption of supplies should be considered and provision to deal with such situations should not be ignored. The emergency exit must be made for release and evacuate livestock quickly if there is an emergency. Consideration should be given to installing fire alarms that can be heard and responded to at any time of the day or night.

6.2.2 Components of a pig housing unit

Building layout and functional areas

The layout of the building should be designed by considering the number of stock and extension scope in the future. The function area should include the adequate space requirement for the pig to eat, drink, rest and exercise. There should be enough space for use of equipment for feed, water, manure removal, treatment and other husbandry procedures. Other operational space requirements for handling, weighing, loading and unloading pigs, breeding, quarantine, examination and treatment of pigs, feed storage, storage for manure and contaminated drainage water, equipment storage, equipment and vehicle repair area, disposal of the carcass should be considered. Additional areas may be needed for an office, restroom, showers and lockers. A lunchroom, animal or equipment cleaning, feed processing, hazardous waste storage, supplies receiving and shipping and vehicle parking may also be needed.

Construction details

Construction should be done as per the pig rearing system and climatic conductions. It is difficult to describe the material utilized and the cost of construction as the price and availability vary globally. The general plan of construction is explained below.

Floor

All floors must be concrete. The floors should be at least 10cm thick, even beneath slatted flooring. The use of steel reinforcement bars or mesh in solid slab floors at grade level is generally a waste of money in livestock buildings. Slatted floors are recommended to minimize water usage for pig bathing and floor washing. No dirt floors should be permitted in any barn area. The floor should slope 4-5% (1:20 to 1:25) toward the waste-collection drain or slatted area. Floor openings and gutters should be sized and spaced to prevent hoof or leg injury of pigs.

Walls and ceilings

Barn roofs should have a minimum slope of 20 and must have a covered ridge opening (1.2 m wide and 0.6 m deep, minimum) along their entire length. Provisions must be made to collect rainwater from the roofs with gutters or concrete drains along the eaves of the barns.Walls and ceilings enclose interior space for security and environmental modification but may be unnecessary or undesirable for some facilities sheltering larger swine and for some climate and weather conditions. The climatic conditions, type of housing and management practices determine the most suitable amount of insulation, moisture permeability and surface finish. Surfaces should be easy to clean and, where necessary, resistant to damage from animal contact and impact.

Corridors and Doors

Corridors need to be wide enough so that animals, personnel and equipment can move around easily. Doors will vary in size and material (metal or wood) according to the function they serve. In an enclosed facility, they should fit tightly within their frames in such a way that pig may not lift it by putting snout under it.

Feed trough

It should provide adequate access to feed for each stage of production. Design and space requirements should be as per the size of the pig using it. Troughs should be able to be easily cleaned to prevent feed accumulation and spoilage. For nurseries, consider the needs of the newly weaned pig and the largest pig which will be in the nursery. The feeder should meet the needs of both animals. Pigs may be fed on boards on the floor the first few days after weaning. Where pigs are fed on a rationed feed level to control intake, it should be ensured that adequate trough space is provided to ensure that all pigs can receive their allocation (table 6.2). Good hygiene is necessary for storage and feeding systems as molds can develop in the stale feed that can have a detrimental effect on pigs.

Table 6.2: Weight of pig and recommended trough space per pig.

Weight of Pig (KG)	*Trough space (cms)*
5	10
10	13
15	15
35	20
60	23
90	28
120	30

Waterers

Waterers should be positioned to ensure pigs have adequate access. Flow rates should be as per the water intake requirements of the pig. Various kinds of waterer options are available including various types of cups and nipple waters. Permanent access to a sufficient quantityof fresh drinking water to all pigs over two weeks of age must be provided. Water requirements (minimum) are given in table 6.3.

Table 6.3 - Minimum daily water requirements for various weights of pig

Weight of Pig (KG)	*Daily requirement (Liters)*	*Minimum Flow rate through nipple drinkers (Liters/min)*
Newly weaned	1.0-1.5	0.3
Up to 20kgs	1.5-2.0	0.5-1.0
20kgs – 40kgs	2.0-5.0	1.0-1.5
Finishing pigs up to 100kgs	5.0-6.0	1.0-1.5
Sows and gilts	5.0-8.0	2.0
Sows and gilts - in lactation	15.0-30.0	2.0
Boars	5.0-15.0	2.0

Drainage

The handling of solid manure, that is to say, manure and bedding can be stacked in wind-rows. Liquid manure is a combination of all the excreta of the pigs and the water coming from leaking drinking nipples, flushing water for floors and water used for flushing other areas. The handling of liquid manure is preferred as it is less labor intensive than the handling of solid manure. Slatted floors are having an advantage as it reduces direct contact between animals and their feces. Under the slatted floor, there must be a deep storage channel for liquid manure which should never be emptied. Regular flushed cleaning of shallow channels under a slatted floor is required. Open channels or wide concrete alleys should be regularly flushed clean. In comparison to the concrete floor, slatted floors are relatively clean and leave the pen dry hence require less labor. The feeding places should be far away from the manure accumulation areas to avoid contact between the animal and his manure. Usually, animals tend to urinate while they drink hence waterers should be placed over the slatted area.

Space Requirement for Different Classes of Pig

Table 6.4: Space Requirement for Different Classes of Pig

Type of animal	*Floor space requirement (m^2 per animal)*		*Maximum number of animals per pen*
	Covered area	Open paddock	
Boar	6.0-7.0	8.8-12.0	Individual pens
Farrowing pen	7.0-9.0	8.8-12.0	Individual pens
Fattener (3-5 months old)	0.9-1.2	0.9-1.2	30
Fattener (above 5 months)	1.3-1.8	1.3-1.8	30
Dry sow/gilt	1.8-2.7	1.4-1.8	3-10

(Source: National Bank for Agriculture and Rural Development)

6.3 Housing requirements of pigs

Environmental and climate requirements are different for different stages of growth. In order to reach their full potential, boars and sows especially need special attention as far as prevention of high ambient temperatures and other stress factors are concerned.The housing requirements of different pigs at different growth stages is as follows.

Boar pen

The boar pen should be non-slippery, cool and well ventilated. Sufficient bedding materials should be placed in the pen. Besides comfort, bedding material prevents the development of bedsores on the shoulders of heavy boars and chafing of hooves against the concrete. The minimum floor area provided should be 7.0 m . The feed trough should be 45-60 cm long, 15-20 cm high and around 50 cm wide. Per day water requirement of the bore is around 10 to 15 liters. High-quality drinking nipples of 1.2 cm in diameter with a flow rate of 2 liter/min should be used. Because boars are alone in their pens they are particularly prone to the effects of temperature variations. The pen should maintain a temperature around 22 C. Pigs do not sweat and they keep their body cool through evaporation. The high temperatures in summer will also affect boar performance i.e. libido, general activity and affect the sperm quality. In hot summer when there is an extremely high temperature, sperm quality will be affected for up to 6–8 weeks. The provision of cooling is recommended. Hence, in hot weather sprinklers are preferable to moistening because moistening only cools the air, while sprinkling wets the pig and causes the skin to cool through evaporation. Pigs are having the habit of urinating and defecating while drinking water hence waterer should be placed in the dunging area. To prevent the feed from getting wet or soiled by urine or feces, the feeding trough has to be placed as far away as possible from the dunging area and the drinking nipple.

Sow pen

The saw pen is usually placed next to the boar pen because the sow has to stay there for four to five weeks and a sow/boar ratio of 1:20 has to be maintained. The saw and boar pen is connected with partitioned where they communicate. The partitioning over the slatted or dunging area is done as pigs tend to defecate while communicating with pigs in adjoining pens. After weaning the saw should be placed in pen for mating. The sows are placed in the pens of about 1.8 m for individual feeding and the pen should be near to boar pen. The sows are kept in the same building as the boar. For this reason, the same temperature and ventilation requirements apply as those for the boar. Temperatures of between 9 C and 22 C are acceptable, with an optimum of 16 C. The relative humidity between 40% and 70% should be maintained. The estimated water requirements of a non-pregnant sow are five liters per day and the required water flow rate two liters per minute. The feeding trough measurements are the same as those for boars.

Dry sow housing

After successful mating, the saw should be separated from the saw pen as they don't require boar anymore. Up to before farrowing they will stay in fully or partially covered yard or may be housed in crates, in a group, or in tethers. Crates are usually closed at the top with metallic rods to prevent the sow from turning around and jumping out. These dry and pregnant saws are grouped in four or five and should be fed individually with partitioning for each saw. The optimum temperature is between 15 and 16 C should be maintained for the dry saw. Water can be provided by drinking nipples or by a flushing system in a continuous feeding trough.

Farrowing pens

Generally, 25 farrowing pens are enough for 100 saw units. The farrowing pen can be constructed in a variety of ways by utilizing the locally available materials to reduce construction costs. It can be made by using metallic pipes or rods. Sufficient space should be provided for easy farrowing and movement of piglets. The pen has a narrow part with width 45-50cm and the wider part with width 70-85cm and constructed at 30-40cm above the floor. The height of the pen should be 50-60cm. The length of the crate is about 2500 mm and includes the feeding trough in the front part. The narrow part at the top prevents the sow from falling when she lies down and gives the piglets a chance to get out of the way when she lies down. The wide part at the bottom of the crate ensures that the sow lies down comfortably and that the piglets have easy access to her nipples. The floor gradient should be towards the manure channel for the free flow of urine and easy cleaning. Optimum temperature maintenance is essential to the sow and her litter and to limit deaths. Piglets require around 32-370C for the first five days. The cold will lower the resistance of piglets against disease. The pen should be disinfected and the saw should be placed one week before the expected date of farrowing to allow time for adjustment to the new surroundings. Sufficient bedding material (sawdust) should be provided. The lactating sow needs about 15 to 30 liters of water per day and the piglets in the region of 0.5 to 1.0 liters per day. A drinking nipple should be placed with an angle of 45 .

Creeping area

It should be 60cm long and 60cm wide and provided with sufficient bedding material (wood say or hay). Piglets cannot produce sufficient heat for the first five days of birth. So the temperature between 32-370C should be maintained during this period. After that, the piglets can produce enough body heat, except during very cold weather. To keep piglets healthy and alive, they should be kept warm. Saw requires less temperature than piglets. It is preferable not to place the creeping pen too close to the sow, because the heat may cause her discomfort and stress. Creep feeder of 10cm height, 15cm width and 25cm long should be placed in creep area which is filled twice or three times a day.

Weaner pen

The system of weaning pigs is different in a different part of the world. The pigs are generally weaned at the early age of 3 weeks or at 5 weeks. In tropics, it is done at 8 weeks. Maintenance of temperature around 25-290C is important in the case of early weaning. If weaning is done at 35 days, a total of 14 weaner pens are required for a 100 sow unit, taking into account that each sow weans on average 2.3 litters per year and that each litter contains an average of 10 piglets. The all-in-all-out system should be applied and there have to be enough pens to allow a cleaning period of seven days. The all-in-all-out pens are designed to accommodate all the litters of the sows that give birth in the same week in an enclosed section of the building when they are being weaned. Afterward they are transferred to a grower unit - all during the same week. All piglets are moved to the grower pens at five weeks. Concrete floor is undesirable for weaner pigs because they chill easily when wet. Several different flooring materials (plastic-coated expanded metal, woven wire, and bare-woven wire) can be used. A newly weaned pig should have a clean, dry, warm environment where waste is removed as quickly as possible. The floor should be totally slatted because the small pig is not trained to use one specific area. For the least stress and best performance, each of the pens should be divided in half, and a feeder should be placed at each end. One litter of seven or eight pigs can be placed in each pen.

Grower and finisher Pen

Weaner pigs are normally moved to the grower pens. At this stage, they weigh around 30 kg. The temperature requirement at this stage ranging between 12 and 180C. Depending on the stage at which the pig is marketed, it will remain in the grower house until it reaches a weight of between 60 kg and 110 kg. Feeding is the basic difference between grower and finisher house. The space requirement in the grower and finisher house is based on the weight of the pigs. The average norm is about 8.5-9 ft per 45 kg, 10-10.5 ft for up to 90 kg and 10.5-14 ft for up to 110 kg live body weight. Manure inside the building can be handled by the use of slatted floors over a manure channel. It has long been recognized that pigs will most frequently defecate in a corner of a pen hence, slatted flooring must be used in each corner of the pen. Wide concrete slats of between 10cm and 12cm and spaced 2cm apart are commonly used. Where two litters of more or less 20 piglets are grouped together from the weaning stage, the group is transferred to the grower pen in its entirety. If the norm for a 100 sow unit applies, as mentioned before, about 20 grower pens are required, each designed to house 20 pigs with a live body weight of between 30 kg and 65 kg. These pens are housed in the same building. After this, each group of 20 pigs is separated into two groups. After the gilts have been taken out of the group, the remaining eight or ten pigs go to the finishing pens where they are kept until they are marketed. Double the number of pens is required for the finishing house. A self-feeder is used for growers, while finishers use a feeding trough allowing 30cm per pig, with a height of 15cm to 20cm and a width of 30cm. Growers and finishers require about five to ten liters of drinking water per day should be provided with drinking nipples.

Manure Disposal

Pigs should be kept in clean, comfortable and healthy surroundings. Wastes must be managed in a manner that will maintain sanitary conditions for the pigs, prevent fly breeding, minimize odors, and protect groundwater quality. Fly eggs will not hatch when manure is completely dry, nor when it is in a liquid flow form. A manure handling, storage, or disposal system must aim at quickly converting manure, urine, and other wastes to a very dry form or a very wet form. The very dry and wet forms also minimize odors. The density of the hog population will help to determine the degree of waste management necessary. The total amount of excreta (feces and urine per day) is about 7.7 kg per 100 kg hog. This is equivalent to a volume of 0.275 cubic feet of space. Swine manure contains nutrients that can support crop production and enhance the soil's chemical and physical properties. The plant nutrients in manure can reduce a producer's fertilizer costs. Thus, manure can be an asset to a pork production operation if its nutrient value is maximized.

Manure management has become a major factor in determining the location and population limits of operations. Poor manure management can result in increased disease in the pigs, odor issues, and declining water quality. Pork producers select a manure handling system based on state regulations as well as factors such as location, size, type, and use of their cropland, the number of animals they have on-site, and the type of animal housing. Solid manure results from holding manure in bedding or by allowing liquid to runoff and should be handled separately. It should be disposed of by spreading in fields. Unbedded solid manure results in a slurry with consistency between a solid and liquid. It is difficult to store and can be picked up by bucket and disposed of by spreading. Liquid manure handling is comparatively easy. It can be handled by a flushing system in which a large volume of water flows from one end down to the slope in the shallow gutter. Mechanical scrapers can also remove manure from open or underslat gutter. Liquid manure can be disposed of by field spreading with tank wagon.

❑❑❑

Chapter 7

The Digestive System of the Pig

—Dr. Awot Teklu, Mr. Tsegay Tkue, Mr. Hailay Kidanu

The pig is a mono-gastric (simple stomach) and non-ruminant like human beings. The digestive system of pig differs from that of ruminants' digestive system found in cattle, sheep and goats as their stomach has four compartments. Due to the difference in their stomach, their feed ingredients differ. In ruminants, the fodder is the major component of their ration but in pigs, concentrates are easier to digest than ruminants' one. Digestion is the break-down of food particles in the digestive tract. The digestive tract is a long tube through which food passes for digestion. When food is broken down into smaller and smaller units as it passes through the digestive tract, it. These small units of food are absorbed as nutrients and undigested food excreted out of the body as feces.

The digestive tract of the pig consists of the mouth, esophagus, stomach, and small and large intestines (figure 7.1).

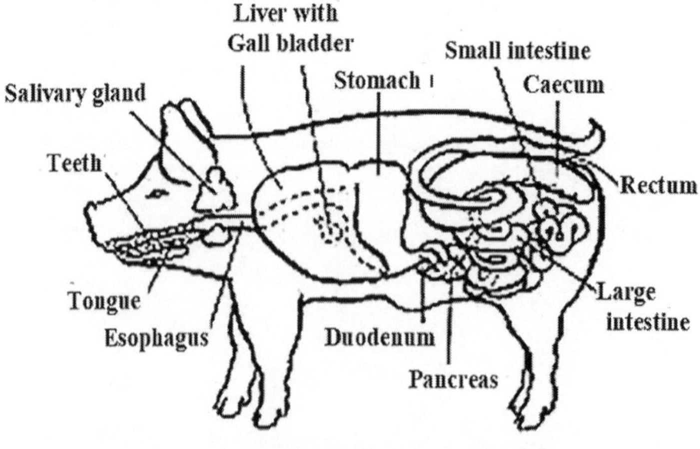

Figure 7.1: Digestive system of the pig

7.1 Digestion and Absorption in Different Part of Digestive System

Mouth and esophagus

The mouth or oral cavity is responsible for the ingestion and the mechanical reduction of food particles with the help of teeth. Teeth grind the feed to reduce the size of the feed particle and increase the surface area. The first action of the chemical breakdown of food occurs when feed is mixed with saliva. There are three main salivary glands i.e. parotid, mandibular and sublingual salivary gland. The saliva secreted from these glands also contains mucous which softens the food. The amount of mucous released depends on the moisture content of the feed. More mucous is secreted when feed is dry and vice versa. Saliva contains the enzyme 'amylase' (although at a very low level) that hydrolyses starch to maltose. The contribution of saliva in digestion is less. After food is mixed with saliva through chewing, it passes to the esophagus through the pharynx. Food pass to the stomach through the esophagus due to contraction and relaxation of the associated muscle. The esophagus terminates with the cardiac valve, which prevents food from passing from the stomach back into the esophagus.

Stomach

The stomach is a muscular organ consists of four regions i.e. esophageal, cardiac, fundic and pyloric. At the entrance of the esophagus into the stomach, the esophageal region is located. No enzyme is secreted in this region. The food is passed from this region to the cardiac region. In the cardiac region, mucous is secreted and mixed with the ingesta. Ingested food then pass to fundic region digestion of food majorly begins (figure 7.2). The major secretions are:

- Hydrochloric acids from gastric glands which reduce the pH up to 1.5 to 2.5 which kills ingested bacteria with feed.
- Pepsinogen is a digestive enzyme that is converted into pepsin in the presence of hydrochloric acid. Pepsin is involved in the breakdown of protein.

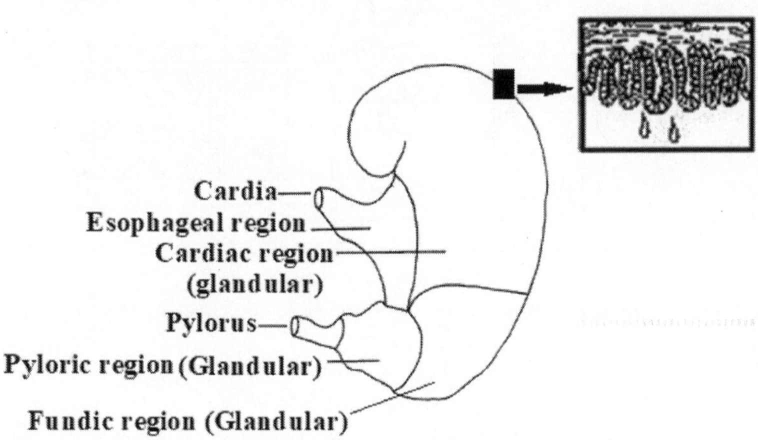

Figure 7.2. Regions of the stomach

Digesta then moves to the pyloric region of the stomach where mucous is secreted to line the digestive membranes to prevent damage from low pH of digesta (also called chyme) while passing to the small intestine. The flow of chime is regulated by the pyloric sphincter which is present at the junction of the pyloric region and the beginning of the small intestine.

Small intestine, pancreas and liver

The organization of the small intestine is complex as it is highly coiled spirally and serves as the major site of nutrient absorption (figure 7.3). It is lined with villi (many tiny finger-like projection) which increases the surface area for absorption. The lining of the small intestine wall secrete enzymes that help in digestion and absorption. The small intestine is divided into three parts i.e. duodenum, jejunum and ileum. The first section is the duodenum where the secretions from the pancreas and liver (gall bladder) are added.

Pancreas

The secretion of the pancreas is exocrine as well as endocrine. It secretes insulin and glucagon to control the sugar level of the body. Exocrine secretions of the pancreas are digestive enzymes and NaHCO3 (Sodium bicarbonate). These digestive enzymes hydrolyse protein, fat and sugar and sodium bicarbonate adds alkalinity of the chime as it has very low pH which may damage the intestinal lining.

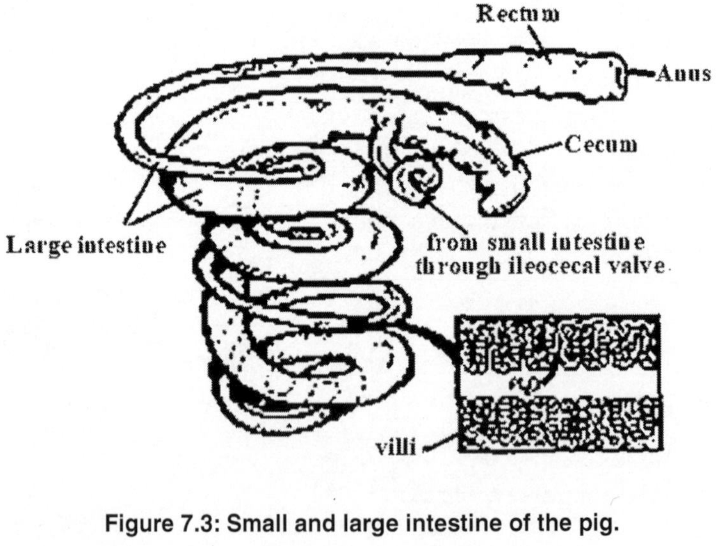

Figure 7.3: Small and large intestine of the pig.

Liver and gall bladder

Gall bladder stores secretion of the liver called bile is responsible for the digestion of fat. It also helps in the absorption of fat-soluble vitamins and cholesterol. The absorption of cholesterol takes place in the lower part of the small intestine and circulated to the liver via portal vein.

Chime then pass to the second part of the small intestine, jejunum where the further breakdown of food and absorption of nutrients takes place. A major portion of food is absorbed in the jejunum and third part of the small intestine, ileum. The absorption is facilitated due to the presence of villi (brush border epithelium). Amino acids and simple sugars are absorbed through villi and taken to the liver via circulatory system. Dietary fat after digestion enters the lymphatic system and via thoracic duct released into circulation.

Large intestine

No enzymatic digestion occurs in the large intestine. Undigested food enters the large intestine through the ileocecal valve. Cecum which is also called the blind gut is located at the beginning of the large intestine. It is having a blind end and ingesta cannot pass through it. It is connected with the colon from where the digesta passes to the rectum and finally excreted out through the anus as feces. The large intestine is basically responsible for the absorption of water. In pigs, limited microbial digestion occurs in the large intestine. Volatile fatty acids form to limited extent by the action of the microbial enzyme and it is absorbed by the large intestine. Vitamin B is synthesized and absorbed in a limited amount in the large intestine.

Chapter 8

Nutrition of Swine

—Dr. Awot Teklu, Dr. Kiros Abebe, Mr. Tsegay Tkue

8.1 Nutrient requirements and feeding of pigs

Like other livestock, swine also require nutrients like water, carbohydrates, fats, protein (amino acids), minerals, and vitamins. Antibiotics, chemotherapeutic agents, and other feed additives are commonly added to swine diets to increase the rate and efficiency of gain and for other purposes, but they are not considered nutrients. National Research Council (NRC) requirements are on a 90% DM basis and for Large White Yorkshire, Landrace, Berkshire, etc. while the Bureau of Indian Standards (BIS) specifications are on a 100% DM basis and for indigenous and improved and crossbred pigs.

Protein and amino acids

Amino acids are supplied by dietary protein. It is required for maintenance, production and reproduction i.e. muscle growth, fetal development in gestating sows, and milk production in lactating sows. Out of 22 amino acids, only 12 are synthesized by the animal while the rest 10 must be added in the diet for normal growth. The 10 dietary essential amino acids for growing pigs are arginine, histidine, isoleucine, leucine, lysine, methionine, phenylalanine, threonine, tryptophan, and valine. Cysteine and tyrosine can meet a portion of the requirement for methionine and phenylalanine, respectively.

The amino acids of greatest practical importance are lysine, tryptophan, threonine, and methionine. The basic grain in most swine ration is maize which is deficient in tryptophan and lysine. The other principal grains for pigs (sorghum, barley, and wheat) are low in lysine and threonine. The first limiting amino acid (essential amino acid found in the smallest quantity in the foodstuff) in soybean meal is methionine.

Animal protein sources are rich in lysine, tryptophan and methionine. The fish meal, however, should not be fed at levels higher than 10% as otherwise objectionable fishy flavor may develop in the pork. Dried blood cells or dried animal plasma are usually deficient in methionine. However, high levels of methionine can depress growth, so methionine should not be added indiscriminately to diets. Milk protein is well balanced in essential amino acids but usually, it is too expensive to be used in swine diets, except for very young pigs.

Clinical signs of amino acid deficiencies or imbalances

The first sign of amino acids deficiency or imbalance is usually a reduction in feed intake accompanied by increased feed wastage, impaired growth and general unthriftiness. Swine can tolerate high intakes of proteins with no ill effects, except occasional mild diarrhea. But large intakes of individual amino acids can lead to a variety of negative syndromes that have been classified as toxicity, antagonism and imbalance, depending on the nature of the effect.

Antagonism commonly occurs among amino acids that are structurally related. An example is a lysine-arginine antagonism. Excessive dietary lysine increases the requirement of arginine. Similarly, the addition of as little as 20 g of leucine to a kg of diet deficient in isoleucine may have a deleterious effect on performance.

Energy requirements

Energy requirements of swine are expressed as the amount of metabolizable energy (ME) per kg diet. ME consists of 94 to 97% DE (average 96%). The loss of energy as gas produced in the digestive tract of swine is usually 0.5 to 1% of DE. ME decreases if protein in the diet is of poor quality. ME also decreases if the excess protein is given to the animal because the amino acids not used for protein synthesis are catabolized and used as a source of energy and nitrogen is excreted as urea. Therefore, as the nitrogen content of the urine increases, ME content of the diet decreases. The energy requirements of pigs are influenced by:

- Their weight (which influences the maintenance requirement),
- Their genetic potential of pig for tissue growth or milk production, and
- The environmental temperature at which they are housed.

The amount of feed consumed by growing pigs fed ad lib is controlled principally by the energy content of the diet. If the energy density of the diet is increased by including supplemental fat, voluntary feed consumption decreases. Pigs fed such a diet will gain weight at a faster rate but the fat in the carcass may increase. If the diet contains excessive amounts of fiber (>5-7%) without commensurate increases in fat, the rate and especially the efficiency of gain are decreased.

Energy requirements of sow

Pregnancy: The sows should be fed and managed to gain a net of 25 kg throughout pregnancy for at least the first 3 or 4 parities. The increase in weight of the placenta and other products of conception should be approximately 20 kg, for a total of 45 kg gestation weight gain of the sow. If pregnant sows are offered feed ad libitum, they will consume more energy than they required for maintenance and the development of the products of conception. Such sows deposit more body fat and protein. Hence it is necessary to limit the energy intake of gestating sows. The energy restriction during gestation has little effect on either litter size or birth weight.

Lactation: Energy requirements during lactation include a requirement of maintenance and a requirement for milk production. DEm for lactating sow is 110 Kcal/kgW0.75/day which is the same as that for the gestating sow. Energy requirements for milk production are 2 Mcal of DE/kg milk (assuming GE of milk 1.3 Mcal DE/kg of milk and 65% efficiency of utilization).

Minerals and vitamins

A common problem of calcium or phosphorus deficit sow is a paralysis of the hind legs known as posterior paralysis. It occurs commonly in high milk-producing sows towards the end of or just after the end of lactation. It has been established that the supplementation of cobalt prevents lesions associated with zinc deficiency. Osteochondrosis, a fault in load-bearing joints is non-inflammatory and involves the cartilage tissue around the end of the bone. Pigs with high porcine somatotropin (PST) levels seem more predisposed toosteochondrosis than with low levels.

Water

Pigs should have free access to water. The amount of water required varies with the type of feed, age, the status of lactation, fever, environmental temperature, high urinary output (as from high salt or protein intake), or diarrhea. For every kg of dry feed, growing pigs usually consume 2-3 kg of water. Lactating sows consume more water because of the high water content of the milk that they produce. Performance and milk production and death may occur if water restriction is severe.

Feeding of Piglets

In addition to sows' milk, creep feeding is essential for piglets for faster growth. The sow's milk (peak at 3 weeks of age) is unable to support the growth of piglets exclusively on milk. Provide a fresh creep feed to the piglets from 7-10 days of age and continue up to 56 days of age at which piglets are weaned from the mother @ 200 g twice a week per piglet. If weaning is practiced at an early age of 3 weeks (Segregated early weaning, SEW) a special pre-starter ration should be used.

Intake of adequate amounts of a creep ration is often a problem that can be overcome by placing the creep feeder in a warm, dry, well-lighted area. Sprinkling feed on the floor or placing it in a shallow pan may help pigs start to eat. Pelleted feeds are usually eaten more readily than meals. Add ferrous sulphate in the creep mixture at 1:9 ratios. Iron dextrin injection (i/m) is to be given on the 4th and 14th day of age to prevent piglet anemia.

NRC (1988) suggested three levels of protein, viz. 24%, 20% and 18% during 1-5 kg, 5-10 kg and 10-20 kg body weight, respectively while BIS (1986) suggested one level of protein (20%) only. Phase feeding, as suggested by NRC, helps the piglets to make rapid gains during early age. All boars are castrated at weaning age except some boars needed for breeding purposes.

Feeding of Pigs

In pigs, fermentative digestion occurs in the caecum and colon. Fermentative products chiefly VFA may meet to 25 to 30% of the maintenance requirements of pigs. An adult pig can handle 3-5 kg of leafy green feeds. Source and levels of fiber besides other nutrients decide the level of fiber in pigs' diet. In growing-fattening pigs, 6-8% CF may be used while the adult's ration may contain 10-12%. Pigs less than 2 to 3 weeks old have insufficient pancreatic amylase and intestinal disaccharidases. Hence after 2 weeks of age only, pigs are to be fed starch-or-cereal-based diets. Afterward only, pigs can utilize fructose and sucrose.

Feeding of growing-finishing pigs

Pigs are fed starter, grower and finisher diets as per the requirement. The CP (%) and ME (Kcal/kg diet) requirements are 18 and 3250, 15 and 3260 and 13 and 3275, respectively (NRC 1988). BIS (1986) specified only three types of feeds for pigs and these are creep/starter diet (rations to be fed up to weaning), pig growth meal (rations to be fed from weaning to 35 kg live weight) and pig finisher/breeding meal (rations to be fed from 35 kg live weight).

After weaning the piglets at 8 weeks of age, the sow should be flushed, i.e. put on a more nutritious ration for a couple of weeks and then mated during the first heat period. Three or four days before farrowing, the ration should be made more laxative through the introduction of more wheat bran. On the day it farrows, gilt/sow should be given plenty of slightly warm water but no feed. On the next day, it can be given 1 to 1.5 kg laxative ration. On the succeeding days, the amount fed can be increased through the gradual introduction of the regular lactation ration so that sow is on full feed in about 7 days after farrowing.

The requirements of the lactating sow are greater than those during the gestation period. A rule of thumb method is to provide daily 2 to 3 kg ration for maintenance plus 0.2 to 0.5 kg for each piglet the sow is nursing. The average birth weight of a LWY piglet is 1.2 kg while a local piglet may weigh 0.7 kg. By 8 weeks of age, Yorkshire pig weighs about 12 kg and it attains a weight of 65 to 70 kg by 6 months of age which is the optimum weight for slaughter for economic pork production in tropics.

8.2 The Efficiency of Feed Conversion in Swine

The amount of feed required for an animal to make a unit gain in weight is called feed efficiency. Pig is superior to beef cattle, goats, or sheep in converting animal feed to human food. Factors that affect feed efficiency:

- Diet should be balanced with an optimum energy protein ratio. It should be balanced with vitamins and minerals.
- Low-quality protein and higher fibre levels in the diet increase the amount of feed nutrients lost in excreta, especially nitrogen.

- Low environmental temperatures reduce the energy available for growth as the animal's maintenance energy requirement is increased hence feed efficiency is decreased.
- Young animals require less feed per unit of gain than older ones. Baby pigs are most efficient in utilizing feed nutrients. The feed efficiencies are 3.13 to 3.35 and 3.82 to 4.13 for growing and finishing LWY pigs. Feed efficiency in swine is 30 to 40% heritable.
- Usually as pigs grow older and become heavier the percentage and amount of fat increases. Decreasing excess fat will increase feed efficiency since fat has about 90% DM whereas lean tissue has about 30% DM.
- Faster gaining animals usually make more efficient gains than slower growing animals.

Steeping: Steeping is the process of making the feed steeped for 9 hours at room temperature and the feed and water ratio is 1: 2.5. Steeping the feed for 9 hours at room temperature reduced the phytate content by 45% and increased the amount of free phosphorus threefold.

Liquid feeding: Liquid feeding usually involves the mixing of predetermined amounts of feed and water prior to or at the time of feeding or feed may be automatically dropped into the water in the feed trough. When properly used, this method can practically eliminate feed dust in the feeding area and minimize waste.

Practical feeding of swine: While formulating ration for a particular class of pigs, the following points should be kept in mind:

- The nutrient requirements for that class of animals.
- The ingredients available and their nutrient levels and limitations.
- Techniques used in formulating diets.

8.3 Nutrient Requirements and Limitations

Determination of the nutrient requirements is essential before formulating a swine ration. The primary concern in formulating a diet is meeting the animal's minimum nutrient requirements. Several nutrients can cause problems when included at high levels. The level of calcium in the diet should not exceed 1.5 times the phosphorus level. Higher levels will result in poorer feed conversion and possibly reduced gains. High levels of salt will reduce feed intake. Salt should not exceed 0.5 percent of the diet. Increased fiber in the ration indicates lower energy content. Fiber should not exceed 5% of the diet for all classes of hogs except possibly gestating sows.

Ingredients and Ingredient Limitations

Once the nutrient requirements have been calculated, select the ingredients. Ingredients can be categorized on the basis of energy sources, amino acid sources, mineral sources, vitamin sources and additives. The grain is the primary source of energy in swine feeds while oilseed meals and animal by-products are the primary sources of amino acids. Corn is the major energy source and soybean meal is the primary protein source in swine ration. There are other alternatives available to both ingredients.

Common problems in swine rations:

The most common problems in swine diets are:

- High calcium levels
- Low phosphorus levels
- High calcium: phosphorus ratios
- Low protein levels

The high calcium levels may stem from excessive calcium in soybean meal (calcium carbonate added as a drying agent). Lower protein levels in the prepared ration may result from poor protein sources or ration formulation errors.

- Nutritional requirements for different stages of pig and deficiency symptoms are given from table 8.1 to 8.12.

Table 8.1: Average chemical composition of ingredients used in swine diets

Ingredient	Metabolizable energy	Protein	Calcium	Phosphorus	Fat	Fiber	Lysine	Methionine &cysteine	Trypto-phan	Threo-+nine
	kcal/lb	Percent			Percent					
Alfalfa meal (dehydrated)	600	17.5	1.40	.26	3.2	23.5	.80	.58	.36	.70
Animal fat	3,590	--	--	--	99.4	--	--	--	--	--
Barley	1,275	11.5	.06	.36	1.8	7	.36	.37	.16	.42
Blood meal	1,200	80	.28	.22	1	1	5.37	2.44	1.02	4.90
Corn (yellow)	1,500	8.2	.01	.24	3.6	2.2	.24	.39	.09	.39
Cottonseed meal (solvent)	1,100	41.7	.20	1.00	2.7	13.4	1.55	1.14	.48	1.32
Defluorinated phosphate	--	--	32.00	18.00	--	--	--	--	--	--
Dicalcium phosphate	--	--	20.00	18.50	--	--	--	--	--	--
Distillers dried grains & solubles, corn	1,270	27	.35	.95	8.0	8.5	.60	1.00	.20	.92
Fish meal (menhaden)	1,200	61.5	5.10	2.98	9.7	.7	4.60	2.50	.71	2.50
Grain sorghum (milo)	1,425	9.8	.02	.27	3.0	2.8	.22	.31	.09	.27
Meat & bone meal	1,100	50.6	8.90	3.93	10.8	2.4	2.50	1.27	.29	1.50
Molasses, cane	1,060	3	.50	.05	--	--	--	--	--	--
Oats	1,200	12	.10	.33	4.0	12.0	.40	.33	.13	.16
Oat goats	1,450	15.8	.08	.43	6.2	2.5	.45	.46	.18	.20
Peanut meal	1,375	52.3	.15	.55	4.1	6.0	1.78	1.26	.55	.49
Skim milk, dried	1,545	33	1.25	1.00	.5	--	2.70	1.20	.45	1.60

Ingredient	Metabolizable energy	Protein	Calcium	Phosphorus	Fat	Fiber	Lysine	Methionine &cysteine	Trypto-phan	Threo-+nine
	kcal/lb	Percent			Percent					
Soybean meal (solvent, hulled)	1,520	49.2	.40	.65	1.5	3.3	3.20	1.55	.63	1.92
Soybean meal (solvent)	1,475	45.6	.50	.71	2.1	5.9	2.88	1.22	.55	1.81
Soybeans (whole cooked)	1,600	38	.25	.58	18.0	5.0	2.40	1.05	.55	1.50
Sunflower meal (extracted w/hulls)	1,044	28.7	.38	.97	2.7	24.8	1.47	2.00	.52	2.13
Wheat	1,500	11.9	.01	.22	1.7	2.8	.35	.34	.12	.32
Wheat bran	890	15.0	.14	1.10	4.1	11.0	.50	.27	.27	.42
Wheat middlings	910	17.1	.10	.88	4.4	7.9	.60	.31	.20	.49
Whey (dried)	1,445	12	.90	.80	.5	--	.80	.40	.13	.89

Table 8.2: Maximum Levels of Ingredients for Swine Diets

	Maximum level % in complete feed				
Ingredient	Starter	Grower-Finisher	Gestation	Lactation	Remarks*
Alfalfa meal-dehydrated	0	5	50	10	A
Animal fat	5	8	8	8	B
Barley	0	80	80	50	C
Blood Meal	5	5	5	5	D
Cottonseed meal	0	5-10	5	5	E
Meat and bone meal	0	5	10	10	D
Oats	10	20	70	15	C
Peanut meal	0	5	5	5	F
Rye	0	20	20	20	G
Tankage	0	5	5	5	D
Wheat bran	0	0	30	10	C
Wheat middling	5	10	30	10	C

Remarks*:

- A. High fiber, low energy but high in B vitamins.
- B. High energy, but can cause feed handling problems when over 8% of the diet.
- C. Low energy, high fiber (7-12% crude fiber).
- D. High protein, but can reduce palatability of the diet.
- E. Low lysine compared to soybean meal; contains gossypol, which is toxic to swine. Can replace up to 50% of the protein from soybean meal.
- F. Low in lysine and methionine; can replace up to 50% of the protein from soybean meal.
- G. Low energy, high fiber, can reduce palatability

Table 8.3: Nutrient Requirements of Swine Allowed Feed Ad libitum (90% DM) (Adapted from NRC 1988).

Intake and performance levels	*Swine Live weight (kg)*				
	1-5	*5-10*	*10-20*	*20-50*	*50-110*
Expected wt. gain g/day	200	250	450	700	820
Expected feed intake, g/day	250	460	950	1900	3110
Expected efficiency, feed/grain	1.25	1.84	2.11	2.71	3.79
Metabolizable energy, Kcal/kg	3220	3240	3250	3260	3275
Protein %	24	20	18	15	13
Indispensable amino acids (important only)					
Lysine %	1.40	1.15	0.95	0.75	0.60
Methionine+cystine%	0.68	0.58	0.48	0.41	0.34
Threonine %	0.80	0.68	0.56	0.48	0.40
Tryptophan %	0.20	0.17	0.14	0.12	0.10
Linoleic acid (%)	0.1	0.1	0.1	0.1	0.1

Table 8.4: Nutrient Requirements of Breeding Swine (Adapted from NRC 1988).

Intake levels	*Breeding gilts, sows & adult boars*	*Lactating gilts and sows*
DE, Kcal /kg diet	3340	3340
ME, Kcal /kg diet	3210	3210
CP%	12	13

Table 8.5: Requirements for Pig Feeds.

S.N.	*Characteristic*	*Requirement*		
		Pig Starter/Creep Feed	*Pig growth Meal*	*Pig Finishing/ Breeding Meal*
1	Moisture content, percent by mass, Max	11.0	11.0	11.0
2	Crude Protein (N2 x 6.25), percent by mass, Min	20.0	18.0	16.0
3	Crude fat or ether extract, percent by mass, Min	2.0	2.0	2.0
4	Crude fibre, percent by mass, Min	5.0	6.0	8.0
5	Total ash, percent by mass, Max	8.0	8.0	8.0
6	Acid insoluble ash, percent by mass, Max	4.0	4.0	4.0
7	Metabolizable energy (Kcal/kg), Min	3360	3170	3170

Note: The values specified for requirements 2 to 6 are on moisture free basis.

Table 8.6: Requirements for Pig Feeds.

S.N.	*Characteristic*	*Requirement*		
		Pig Starter/Creep Feed	*Pig growth Meal*	*Pig Finishing/ Breeding Meal*
1	Niacin, mg/kg	17	14	10
2	Pantothenic acid, mg/kg	11	10	10
3	Riboflavin, mg/kg	3	2.4	2.2
4	Vitamin B12 activity, _g/kg	15	11	11
5	Vitamin A, IU/kg	1700	1300	1300
6	Vitamin D, IU/kg	190	180	130

Table 8.7: Nutrient Requirements of Swine Allowed Feed Ad libitum (90% DM) (Adapted from NRC 1988).

Intake and performance levels	*Swine Live weight (kg)*				
	1-5	*5-10*	*10-20*	*20-50*	*50-110*
Expected wt. gain g/day	200	250	450	700	820
Expected feed intake, g/day	250	460	950	1900	3110
Expected efficiency, feed/grain	1.25	1.84	2.11	2.71	3.79
Metabolizable energy, Kcal/kg	3220	3240	3250	3260	3275
Protein %	24	20	18	15	13

Indispensable amino acids (important only)					
Lysine %	1.40	1.15	0.95	0.75	0.60
Methionine+cystine%	0.68	0.58	0.48	0.41	0.34
Threonine %	0.80	0.68	0.56	0.48	0.40
Tryptophan %	0.20	0.17	0.14	0.12	0.10
Linoleic acid (%)	0.1	0.1	0.1	0.1	0.1

Table 8.8: Nutrient Requirements of Breeding Swine (Adapted from NRC 1988).

Intake levels	*Breeding gilts, sows & adult boars*	*Lactating gilts and sows*
DE, Kcal /kg diet	3340	3340
ME, Kcal /kg diet	3210	3210
CP%	12	13

Table 8.9: Requirements for Pig Feeds.

S.N.	*Characteristic*	*Requirement*		
		Pig Starter/ Creep Feed	*Pig growth* Meal	*Pig Finishing/* Breeding meal
1	Moisture content, percent by mass, Max	11.0	11.0	11.0
2	Crude Protein (N2 x 6.25), percent by mass, Min	20.0	18.0	16.0
3	Crude fat or ether extract, percent by mass, Min	2.0	2.0	2.0
4	Crude fibre, percent by mass, Min	5.0	6.0	8.0
5	Total ash, percent by mass, Max	8.0	8.0	8.0
6	Acid insoluble ash, percent by mass, Max	4.0	4.0	4.0
7	Metabolizable energy (Kcal/kg), Min	3360	3170	3170

Table 8.10: Requirements for Pig Feeds.

S.N.	*Characteristic*	*Requirement*		
		Pig Starter/ Creep Feed	*Pig growth* Meal	*Pig Finishing/* Breeding meal
1	Niacin, mg/kg	17	14	10
2	Pantothenic acid, mg/kg	11	10	10
3	Riboflavin, mg/kg	3	2.4	2.2
4	Vitamin B12 activity, g/kg	15	11	11
5	Vitamin A, IU/kg	1700	1300	1300
6	Vitamin D, IU/kg	190	180	130

Table 8.11: Examples of Starter, Grower and Finisher Diets for Pigs (% Composition) (To meet the Nutrient Requirements as specified by BIS, 1986)

Feedstuff	*Creep/Starter diets CP 20% ME 3370 Kcal/kg on DMB CP 17.8% ME 3000 Kcal/kg on 89% DM*	*Grower diets CP 18% ME 3170 Kcal/kg on DMB CP 16.2% ME 2850 Kcal/kg on 89% DM*	*Finisher diets CP 16% ME 3170 Kcal/kg on DMB CP 14.4% ME 2850 Kcal/kg on 89% DM*
Maize	70 60 - -	52 55 - -	57 - -
Jowar	- - 60 -	- - 55 -	- 57 -
Bajra	- - - 60	- - - 55	- - 57
GNC (exp)	20 20 16 18	15 13 13 11	8 8 6
DORB	- 8 9 5	25 23 21.5 20	28 26.5 25
Fish meal	7.5 10 10 10	6 7 7 7	5 5 5
Mineral mixture with salt	2.5 2.0 2.0 2.0	2 2 2 2	2 2 2
Vegetable oil/Animal fat	- - 3.0 5.0	- - 1.5 5	- 1.5 5
Vitamins A, B2,D3------------------25 g/100kg ------------------			
Vitamin 'B' complex ------------------25g/100kg--------------------			

Table 8.12: Minerals, clinical signs of deficiencies and excesses:

Mineral	*Signs of Deficiency*	*Signs of Excess*
Calcium	Agalactia Depressed milk yield, *Fractures, *Hypocalcaemia, Osteomalacia, *Osteoporosis, *Posterior paralysis in sows, *Rickets	Changes in bone formation if zinc is low (parakeratosis) more than 1% may cause problems. Reduced strength of bone
Copper	Leg weakness, Loose faeces if suddenly withdrawn	*Jaundice 200-600g/tonne, Haemorrhage, Death
Iodine	Enlarged thyroid glands, Reproductive failure, Weak hairless pigs at birth	Rare> 800mg/kg
Iron	*Anaemic, *Increased respiration, More prone to piglet diseases, Poor Growth, Pale skin	Death in piglets deficient in vitamin E, Muscle degeneration> 5000 mg/kg
Magnesium	Infertility Rare Poor growth weak joints	Loose faeces>0.5% in diet
Manganese	Infertility Rare Lameness Poor Growth Weak piglets	In appetence>2000ppm
Phosphorus	Poor growth, *Rickets, See calcium also Soft bones	Changes in bone formation, Posterior paralysis in sows
Potassium	Anorexia Rare, Heart malfunction, In coordination, Poor growth, More prone to disease	Loose faeces>1.2% in diet
Pyridoxine (B6)	Poor growth	Unknown
Riboflavin (B2)	Infertility, Weak piglets	Unknown
Thiamine (B1)	Poor appetite and growth, Sudden death	Unknown

Vitamin A	Rare but reports of:	*Epiphyseal plate changes, *Increased incidence of OCD, *Increased requirements for vitamin E, Joint pain, *Leg weakness, *Mulberry heart disease
Vitamin D3	Infertility, In coordination, Poor bone growth, Poor sight, Congenital defects, born blind	Calcification of soft tissues
Vitamin E	Fractures, Lameness, Rickets, Rubbery bones or osteomalcia, Swollen joints	
(Mulberry Heart Disease)	Agalactia, Discoloration of fat, *Gastric ulcers, *Liver, heart and muscle changes, MMA syndrome. Edema disease, Porcine stress syndrome, *Predisposition to: APP, E. coli diarrhea, Respiratory disease, Swine dysentery, *Reduced immune responses, Sudden death, Udder edema	Unknown
Vitamin K	Enhances warfarin poisoning, Poor blood clotting	

Nursing Pigs

A practical goal for feeding the nursing pig is to shift young pigs from liquid to dry food. After three weeks of age, pigs should begin to consume enough creep feed to improve weaning weights and post-weaning growth. The common preparation is given in table-8.13.

Table 8.13: Percent composition of creep feed

Percent composition of creep feed	
Ingredients	*Parts*
Maize/broken wheat	40.0
Barley/Jowar	33.5
Groundnut cake/soybean meal	16.0
Fish meal/fish meal and meat meal (50:50)	8.0
Mineral mixture	2.0
Common salt	0.5

Weaned nursery pigs

This production phase is severely affected by inadequate housing, management and nutrition. Under these conditions, the pigs usually go through a period of little or no growth for seven to 14 days after weaning (post-weaning lag). With proper nutrition, the setback suffered by the pigs can however be reduced. Good nutritional management includes feeding a diet containing high quality, palatable ingredients with the proper nutrient levels and proper feeding methods. Dried whole whey, fish meal, porcine plasma, dried whole blood, soy protein concentrates or isolates and blends of these products are digestible sources of important nutrients. After the pigs have learned to eat a creep diet before weaning, the same diet used in the nursery will encourage the pig to eat and will reduce the post-weaning lag

Growing-finishing pigs

The growing-finishing pig consumes more feed and at this stage feed efficiency and savings are higher. One should select the most economical protein and energy sources and maintain a proper calcium-phosphorus balance. The goal is to reduce feed costs per unit of gain while maintaining rapid daily gains and acceptable carcass quality. However, while feeding a pig that has superior genetic capabilities for the growth of lean tissues, the requirements for nutrients may increase very dramatically. The growing-finishing pig can be fed alternate energy sources such as grain sorghum, barley, wheat, fat and a variety of by-product feedstuffs. The growing-finishing pig can adapt to new feedstuffs rapidly.

❑❑❑

Chapter 9

Reproductive System of Boar

—Dr. Gebregiorgis Ashebir

9.1 The reproductive tract of adult boar

The reproductive tract of adult boar consists of scrotum, testicles, epididymis, the duct system, penis and a number of accessory sex glands (figure 9.1).

Scrotum

It is a pouch or saclike structure in the external body cavity in which testes are present. It is responsible for the protection of the testes and also the external cremaster and tunica dartos muscles of the scrotum play a major role in temperature regulation of the testes by moving them closer to the body during cold weather and farther away from the body wall warm weather. The temperature of testicles is thus 1-70 C lower than body temperature. Both muscles have an abundant supply of nerve fibers that respond to temperature sensors located in the central nervous system. Because boars do not have pendulous testicles like bulls, the tunica dartos is more important than the cremaster muscle in the regulation of testicular temperature. As compared to other farm animals the thermos-regulation mechanism of testes is least developed in boars as they are located sub-anal in position.

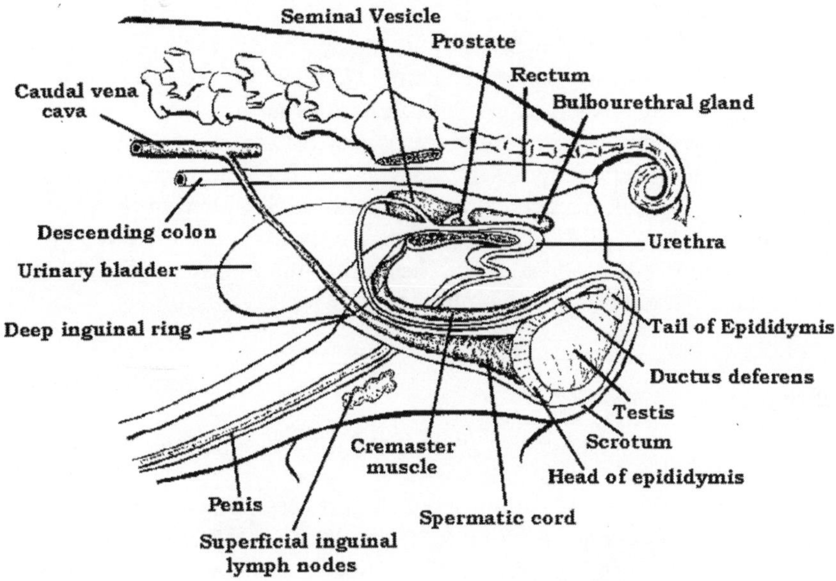

Figure 9.1: Boar reproductive system

Testicles

The testes are developed in the abdomen in the fetal stage and both the testes descend to the scrotal sac at birth or immediately before birth. If one or both testicles fail to descend in the scrotal sac, it results in cryptorchidism. This condition impairs spermatogenesis due to impairing the thermal environment of testes but they are capable of full endocrine function. The primary function of testes is spermatogenesis and production of the male sex hormone, testosterone.

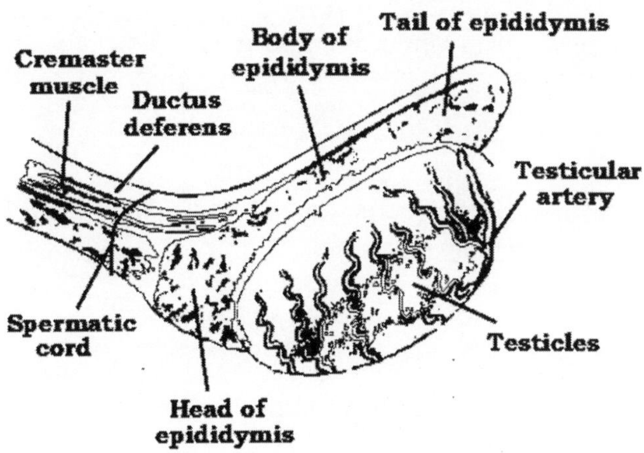

Figure 9.2: Testicle, epididymis, and spermatic cord of the boar

The testis is enclosed in the tunica albuginea surrounded by another tough tunic, the tunica vaginalis (figure 9.2). Sperm is formed in the seminiferous tubules which are a convoluted networks of ducts. The lumen of seminiferous tubules are lined by specialized Sertoli cells which are responsible for the maturation of spermatozoa and production of the hormone. Interstitial cells of Leydig, blood and lymph vessels and nerves are located in between the seminiferous tubules. The sperm is then stored in rete testis which is a collecting duct lined with cuboidal epithelium. The supporting connective tissue joins centrally forming a fibrous cord, the mediastinum testis. During spermatogenesis, spermatozoa leave the seminiferous tubules and enter the rete testis during their passage into the epididymis.

Epididymis

The rete testes exit the boar testicle at the bottom and enter the storage and maturation tube, called the epididymis which is tightly adhered to the outside of the testicle. The epididymis is highly coiled and forms three sections, the caput (head), carpus (body) and the cauda (tail) epididymis. The epididymis is the site for maturation and storage of spermatozoa. Spermatozoa present in the head are neither motile nor fertile. They moved to the body of epididymis due to the flow of rete fluid, ciliated epithelial lining and contraction of the circular layer of muscle.

Vas Deferens and urethra

The vas deferens leaves the testicle to become part of the spermatic cord. It is a thick and heavily muscled tube. They transport the sperm from the tail of the epididymis to the pelvic urethra. The two vas deferens connect with each other and merge into a single tube called the pelvic urethra at the neck of the bladder. The pelvic urethra continues further and passes through the center of the penis where it is known as the penile urethra. The functions of the urethra are to transport both urine and semen. Relaxation of voluntary muscle allows urine to enter into the urethra. Relaxation of this muscle is prevented during erection and ejaculation by the nervous system in order to prevent urine from entering into the semen. Fluids are added to sperm in the pelvic urethra during the process of ejaculation.

9.2 Accessory Sex Glands

Adjacent to the pelvic urethra is three secondary sex glands, the vesicular glands or seminal vesicles; the prostate gland; and the bulbourethral glands. These glands are not essential for fertility but their secretions add substances to the ejaculate that serve to increase volume, protect sperm cells, and provide nutrients needed for ensuring sperm fertility.

Seminal vesicles: It is present lateral to the terminal portion of each vas deferens. These are the largest accessory sex gland. In the boar, they are large, lobulated and relatively diffuse. Their secretion constitutes 15-25% of the fluid volume of bore semen. The secretion has a high level of fructose and citric acid as well as inositol, ergothioneine, several amino acids and glyceryl phosphoroyl choline. Most of these compounds are used as energy substrates by ejaculated spermatozoa.

Prostate gland: It is the smallest accessory sex gland. It is located between the seminal vesicle and the Cowper's gland. A major portion of this gland is embedded in the muscle layer surrounding the pelvic urethra. The secretion of the prostate gland produces thick fluid which is primarily alkaline and contains calcium, acid phosphatase and fibrinolysin. This secretion neutralizes the acidic vaginal secretion. The characteristics odour in semen is due to prostate secretion.

Bulbourethral glands: They are also called the Cowper's gland. These are of intermediate size and long cylindrical glands located on either side of the pelvic urethra near the ischial arch of the pelvis. Secretion of this gland gel-like lubricant material (similar to saliva) which clears the urethra with traces of urine prior to ejaculation. It also lubricates the vulva before vulvar secretion starts flowing. In boar, this gland is well developed.

Penis

The final structure of the boar's urogenital system for the transfer of sperm into the female is the penile urethra. It is a tube-like structure within the penis that opens into the glans penis which is spiral (counter-clockwise). The boar penis is composed of tough fibro-elastic tissue supplied with blood and nerves. During erection blood is pumped in to the boar penis and it extended through an opening called the prepuce located on the abdomen. During normal state, the penis is retracted and forms a characteristic "S" fold called the sigmoid flexure and the free end of the penis resides in the prepuce (figure 9.3). The erectile and non-erectile penis of boar are shown in figure 9.4.

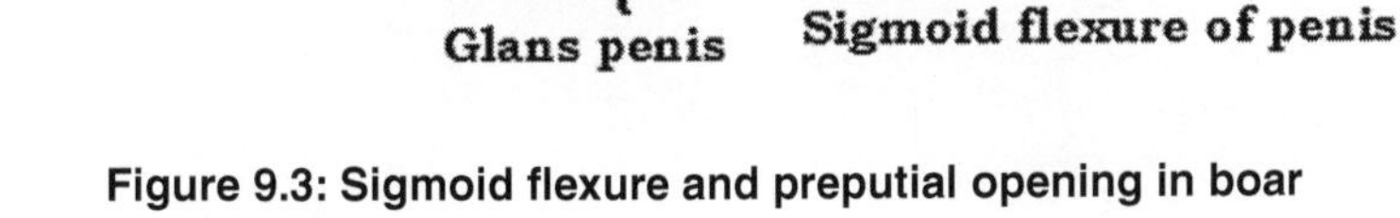

Figure 9.3: Sigmoid flexure and preputial opening in boar

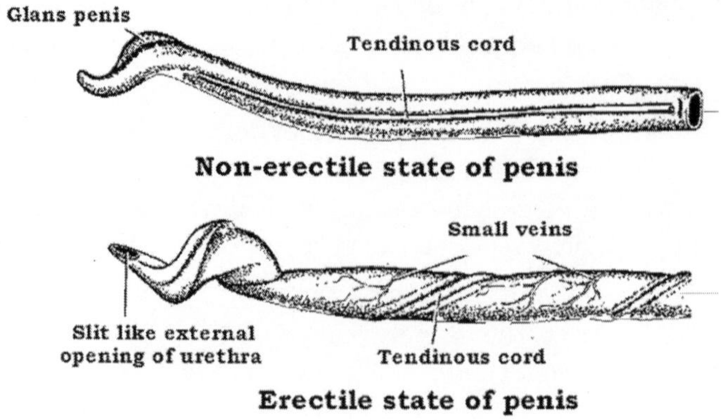

Figure 9.4: Erectile and non-erectile penis of boar.

Near the end of the prepuce is a diverticulum called the preputial sac. Urine, semen and secreted fluid collect in this sac. Contents of the preputial sac are often expelled during the detection of estrus or natural matings and often believed to be the source of the odor associated with mature boars.

❑❑❑

Chapter 10

Reproductive Physiology of Boars

—**Dr. Berihu Gebrekidan**

Reproductive performance of the breeding herd is the major contributing factor for herd productivity. The breeding herd of a farm is dominated by sows and gilts. Boar constitutes 5-10% of the breeding population but it contributes half of the genetic make-up of their progenies. Hence, its contribution should not be ignored. It is important to know the determinants of reproductive performance and boar is one of the significant determinants as it is used for natural service and source of semen for artificial insemination.

10.1 Physiological maturity in boars

Physiological maturation in boars after birth is an ongoing process. The pre-pubertal boar's penis lacks sigmoid flexure. It is attached to the preputial lining with the penile frenulum. The growth of the penis occurs with the influence of testosterone. At this stage, mounting activity in boar increases and these activities lead to sigmoid flexure development and breakdown of the frenulum. At three months of age, there is a rapid increase in the testes to bodyweight ratio. Sperm appears in the seminiferous tubule first time at the age of around four years. At this stage, penile erection can be accomplished in an immature boar. Puberty begins between 5-6 months of age and sperm are present in the ejaculate. Sexual maturity in boars attained at 7-9 months of age depending on the breed. Before sexual maturity, spermatozoa may present in epididymis but adequate libido for mating and ejaculation is lacking.

10.2 Hypothalamus and Pituitary Gland

The brain gathers internal signals from within the body and external cues from the environment and regulates physiological and behavioral functions associated with reproduction. The pituitary gland secretes luteinizing hormone (LH) and follicle-stimulating hormone (FSH) which are responsible for regulating testicular function. Production of these two hormones is controlled by gonadotropin-releasing hormone (GnRH) released from the hypothalamus. The release of GnRH depends on age, weight, the season of the year, nutritional level, environmental temperature, and reproductive status of the testes. These factors individually or collectively influence GnRH and ultimately influence the amount of FSH and LH released into the bloodstream to alter the activity of the testicles.

10.3 Gonadal endocrine activities

The two principal endocrine cells in testes are Leydig cells and Sertoli cells. Production of androgen (primarily testosterone) from Leydig cells is stimulated by luteinizing hormone. Testosterone is essential for normal sperm production. It is also responsible for the maintenance of the accessory sex glands and is involved with libido. Sexually excited boars chomp their jaws, eliciting the production of copious quantities of foamy saliva containing pheromones that stimulate sexual receptivity in estral gilts and sows. Sertoli cell function is regulated primarily by FSH (figure 10.1). Sertoli cells are the only somatic cells found in the seminiferous epithelium and are responsible for the production of inhibin and androgen binding protein which converts testosterone to dihydrotestosterone and estrogen. Inhibin provides the necessary feedback to the anterior pituitary to regulate FSH secretion. Estrogen is present in high quantity in boar's semen which is produced by Sertoli cells, which changes testosterone to estrogen via the aromatase enzyme. Sexual behavior is influenced by estrogen. Estrogen also controls sperm maturation in the epididymis.

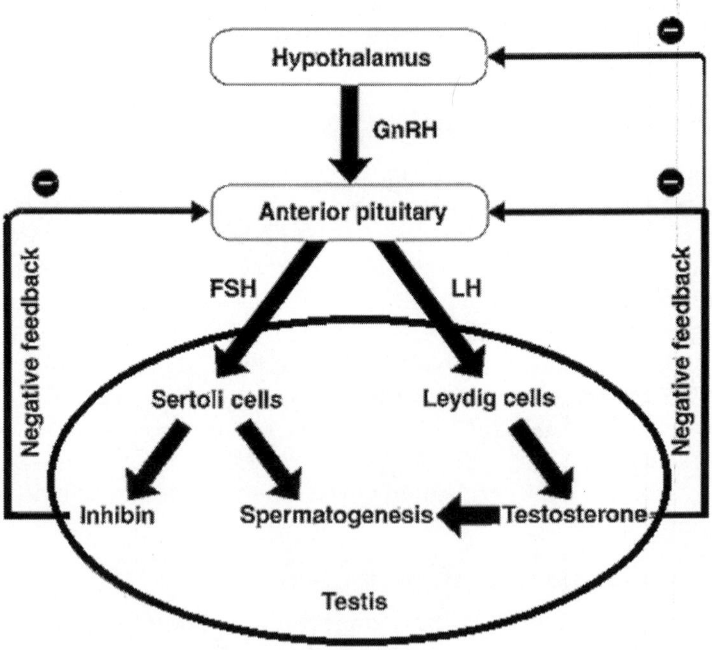

Figure 10.1: Gonadal endocrine activities in male pig.

10.4 Spermatogenesis

Spermatogenesis is a continuous process after puberty is attained. It is divided into spermatocytogenesis and spermiogenesis. Spermatocytogenesis is a multiplication stage involving the mitotic division of spermatogonia and produces primary spermatocyte which undergoes meiosis to produce haploid spermatids known as secondary spermatocytes (figure 10.2 and 10.3). LH plays a more active role than FSH in spermatocytogenesis in spermatocytogenesis. Spermiogenesis refers to the maturational phase of development where haploid spermatids undergo morphologic transformations to become fully differentiated spermatozoa. FSH is the main hormone involved with spermiogenesis.

Spermatozoa then release into the lumen of seminiferous tubules and then undergo a final process of maturation in the epididymis in order to acquire motility and potential fertility. The tail of the epididymis also stores spermatozoa until the time of ejaculation. Spermatogenesis takes around five weeks in the boar, with an additional 9 to 12 days for maturation in epididymis before becoming the fertile gametes emitted during ejaculation.

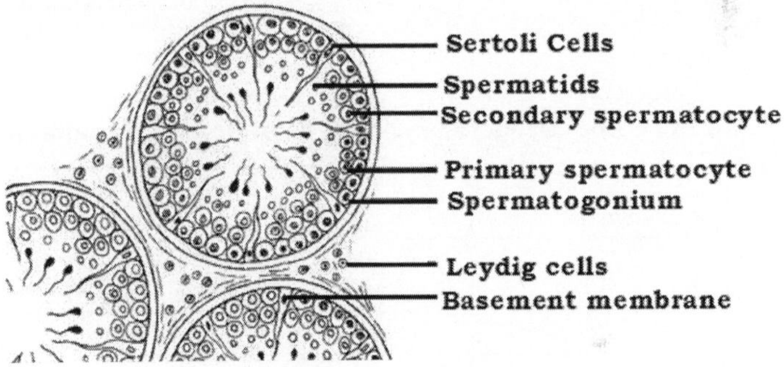

Figure 10.2: Cross-section of the testis.

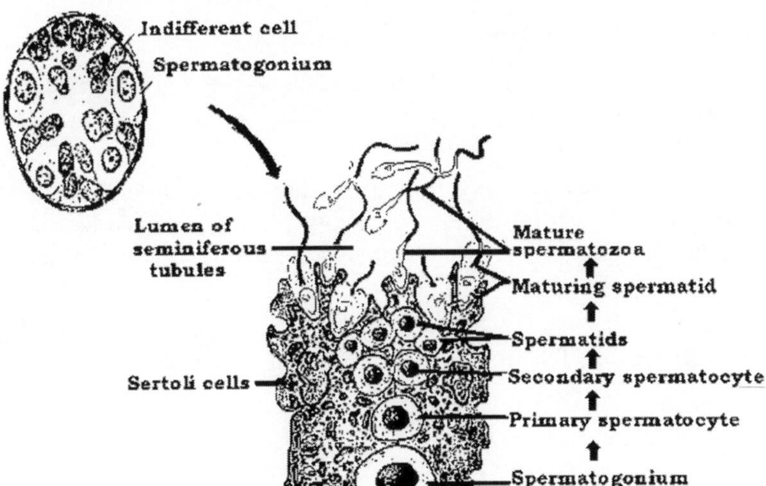

Figure 10.3: Seminiferous tubules.

10.5 Sexual Behaviour of boar

Mounting activity is a very common in males and females even at very early age of one month. But mounting accompanied by erection can be seen after 4 months of age. Ejaculation in boar with a normal concentration of fertile spermatozoa will occur at 6-8 months of age. The erection of the penis is caused by sexual stimulation which causes dilatation of arteries supplying the sinuses of the penis. Testosterone is mainly responsible for the sex drive or libido. On the introduction of the sow, boar approaches her with characteristics grunting sound. Boar will chase the escaping sow with continue grunting sound and grinding of teeth with foaming saliva. If the sow standstill, the boar may nose her flank quite forcefully, sniff the anogenital region and her head, and then attempt to mount. The receptive saw stands immobile with arched back and erected ears and after mounting by boar mating will occur. Ejaculation is indicated by tightening and relaxing of the anal sphincter and should last at least 3 minutes otherwise mating is considered doubtful. The copulation is completed by dismounting.

The ratio of boars to females depends upon age, genetics, libido, season, health and type of mating. The general guideline for the uses of boar is presented in table 10.1.

Table 10.1: Boar Usage Based on Type of Breeding program

Age of boar (months)	*Collection of semen (AI program)*	*Natural mating*		
		Mating/Day	*Total Mating/ week*	*Pen mating (No. of Females/month)*
6-8	1 time/week	1	4	Up to 8
8-12	1-2 times/week	1	5-7	8-10
More than 12	More than 4 times/2 weeks	2	8-10	10-12

10.6 Factors Influencing Semen Quality

To achieve fertilization, the male and female gamete needs to be fertile and exposed to each other in the optimal environment. Some of the important factors influencing semen quality are:

Breed: The study showed that different breeds are having variations in ejaculate volume, concentration, motility and even percent of live/dead cells. German landrace, large white and Yorkshire boars have higher sperm counts than Pietrain and Duroc boars.

Testicular circumference: This is an indicator of the size of the testis. Higher the testicular circumference, the more the testicular size which produces more ejaculate volume.

Age of boar: The size of the testes continues to grow after puberty and leads to an increase in spermatogenic output. This is the reason that to maximize fertility, boars less than 1 year of age should be collected no more than one time per week and boars over 1 year of age can be collected up to two times per week. In older boars, more than 3-4 years of age, sperm abnormality increases which lowers the pregnancy rate and litter size.

Housing: The type of housing for mature boars may affect boar health and indirectly affect semen quality by bacterial contamination. Group housing of growing boars enhances reproductive performance like libido and ejaculate volumes which decreases when pigs are reared in physical isolation from other males or females.

Nutrition: Nutritional restriction below maintenance have a negative effect on sperm output and libido but does not seem to affect sperm motility. The deficiency of protein in diet will affect boar libido and sperm output.

Temperature: Low temperatures are not a great problem for boar fertility but the problem enhanced when temperatures dip below -10 C (14 F). Elevated temperature Temperatures above 85 F reduce both sperm production and motility of ejaculated sperm for up to 2 months. If the temperature further elevated to 95 F for 3 days will lead to increase abnormality in the ejaculate.

Back fat: In some studies, the association of back fat with total sperm motility seemed to be dependent on the storage duration of extended semen. From day 0 to day 2 of storage boars had higher sperm motility when having higher back fat. From day 3 to day 4, a negative association of semen resistance to storage to back fat is observed.

Light: Association of the duration of light on the quality and quantity of semen produced in boar is controversial. Some experiment shows that if boars kept under natural light plus artificial light supplementation to maintain constantly 15 h of light/day from 11 weeks of age until puberty had a rapid sexual maturation with higher libido than boars receiving only natural light during that period.

❒❒❒

Chapter 11

Reproductive System of Sows

—Dr. Berihu Gebrekidan & Dr. Gebregiorgis Ashebir

11.1 Female Reproductive System

In order to achieve optimal reproductive performance, an understanding of the sow's reproductive system is highly essential. Reproductive success is primarily measured by pigs produced per sow per year and is dependent upon both farrowing rate and litter size.

The female reproductive tract of the pig is composed of paired ovaries, oviducts, uterine horns, a single cervix, a vagina and the external genitalia called the vulva. These structures are supported by the broad ligament and hang loosely suspended below and parallel to the rectum in the pelvic cavity and lower abdomen (11.1).

The female reproductive system has the following basic functions

- To produce ova (eggs)
- To facilitate fertilization of ova.
- Provide environment for embryo and fetus to develop
- Give birth to a fetus
- Recycle to become pregnant again
- Provide nourishment to young.

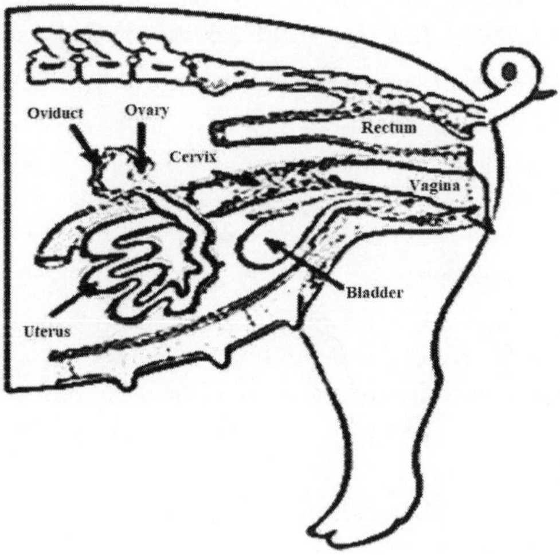

Figure 11.1: The reproductive tract of the sow.

Ovaries

The primary organs of the reproduction are the ovaries whose main functions are the production of the female reproductive cells, the egg or ovum and productions of two hormones, estrogen and progesterone. Ovaries are paired organs located on each side of the uterus in relation to the lateral wall of the pelvis. The actual position is variable depending on the animal, its age, parity, etc. They are usually oval or mulberry-like appearance due to the multiple follicles/corpus luteum present. They weigh 3.5-10 gm and are situated 2.5-5 cm behind the kidneys near the lateral margin of the pelvic inlet. The left ovary is more functional than the right ovary. The anterior (cranial) portion of the broad ligament attached to and supports the ovary and is called the mesovarium. The mesovarium carries the blood and the lymphatic vessels and nerves which supplies the ovary and forms the hilus of the ovary. The second supportive ligament, the utero-ovarian ligament attaches the ovary to the uterus. This utero-ovarian ligament is sometimes called the proper ligament of the ovary and is not acutely part of the broad ligament. The free surface of the ovary is physiologically active where follicles and corpus luteum develops. The mesovarian and uterovarian ligaments form a bursa-like pouch called the ovarian bursa. The sow ovaries are almost completely covered in the bursa. Each ovary is surrounded by a thin membrane called the infundibulum which acts as a funnel to collect ova.

The ovary is covered by the outermost single layer of cuboidal cells called the germinal epithelium. This layer has no function relating to the production of the germinal cells and is thus erroneously named. Beneath the germinal epithelium is the tunica albuginea, a connective tissue composed of fewer cells and closely packed fibers. Beneath the tunica albuginea is the ovarian cortex, which contains the follicles and corpus luteum in various stages of development or regression. Many fibroblasts, some collagen and reticular fibers, blood vessels, nerves, lymphatic vessels and smooth muscle fibers form the connective tissue of the ovarian cortex.

The central part of the ovary is called the ovarian medulla. The medulla houses the vasculature, nerves and the lymphatics and is composed of dense connective tissue.

Within the ovary are follicles in different stages of development:

- A primary follicle is a germ cell surrounded by a single layer of follicular cells. They are located in the parenchyma and seen in groups called egg nests
- Secondary follicles – potential ovum surrounded by two or more layers of follicular cells
- Tertiary Follicle- Development of an antrum (cavity) formed by the collection of fluid between the follicular cells separating them. Antrum filled with liquor folliculi and rich in estrogen. The mature tertiary follicle which appears as a fluid-filled blister on the surface of the ovary is called the Graafian follicle.
- Graafian follicle: In the Graafian follicle, the outermost fibrous cell layer is the theca externa. Inside this layer is the theca interna. Both cell layers are supplied with blood by a capillary network. The basement membrane separates theca interna from the granulosa cells and prevents entry of the vascular system into these cells. The granulosa cells surround the antrum containing liquor folliculi. The cumulus oophorus is located on one side of the antrum. The potential ovum rests upon the discus proligenous. Granulosa cells surrounding and in immediate contact with the ovum are called corona radiata. Both the theca cells and granulosa cells are involved in the production of estrogen.

Oviduct (Salphinx, Egg tube, fallopian tube, Tunnel of love)

The oviducts are a pair of tortuous, narrow tubes suspended in the mesosalphinx, a peritoneal fold from the lateral layer of the broad ligament. They are about 6 to 10 inches long and about 3mm in diameter extending from the ovary to the uterine horn. The oviduct may be divided into four functional segments –the fringe –likefimbriae; the funnel-shaped structure opening adjacent to the ovary-the infundibulum; the more dilated ampulla and the narrow portion of the oviduct connecting the oviduct with the uterine lumen-the isthmus.

The opening of the infundibulum, Ostium tubae abdominale, lies in the center of a fringe of irregular processes, that forms the extremity of the oviduct, the fimbriae. The opening of the isthmus into the uterus is called Osteum tubae uterinum. The fimbriae greatly increase the surface area of the infundibulum and cause it to glide or slip over the entire surface of the ovary near the time of ovulation. The fimbriae are unattached except at one point at the upper pole of the ovary, which also assures close approximation of the fimbriae and ovarian surface. The infundibulum leads directly into a thick portion of the oviduct called the ampulla. The ampulla occupies one- half or more of the oviductal length and merges with the isthmus of the oviduct. The junction between ampulla and isthmus is called ampullary isthemic junction. The isthmus is smaller in diameter than the ampulla. It is connected directly to the uterus and the point of juncture is called the uterotubal junction. This junction is guarded by a long finger-like mucosal process and serves as a major barrier to sperm transport and thus preventing polyspermy.

The wall of the oviduct consists of the mucosa, the muscularis and the outer serous coat. The oviductal mucosa is made of primary, secondary and tertiary folds. The mucosa in the ampulla is thrown into high, branched folds that decrease in height toward the isthmus and become low ridges in the uterotubal junction. The mucosa consists of the surface columnar epithelial cells, muscle fibres and an underlying connective tissue containing fine blood and lymph vessels. The epithelium contains ciliated and non-cilated cells or secretory cells together with `peg cells' (depleted secretary cells). The percentage of ciliated cells decreases gradually in the ampulla toward the isthmus and reaches a maximum in the fimbriae and infundibulum. So the ciliated cells are more abundant where the egg is picked up from the ovarian surface whereas secretory cells are abundant where luminal fluids are needed as a medium for the interaction of egg and spermatozoa. The oviductal epithelium undergoes morphologic and cytologic changes during the estrous cycle.

The muscularis consists of an inner layer of circular or spiral muscle fibers and an outer layer of longitudinal bundles. The thickness of the oviductal musculature increases from the ovarian to the uterine end. The serosa consists of connective tissue and an external coat formed from the peritoneum.

Adrenergic innervation is prominent in the musculature of the isthmus and at the ampullary isthmic junction and these dense adrenergic innervation permits the isthmus to act as a physiologic sphincter which may be important for regulating egg transport.

Functions of the oviduct

1. Captures and transports the ovulated eggs from the ovarian surface to the fertilization site
2. Conveys the egg and spermatozoa in opposite direction, almost simultaneously
3. Sperm capacitation, fertilization and embryo cleavage occur in the oviduct
4. Transport of the early embryo to the uterus
5. The oviduct provides an optimal environment that is both nutritive and protective for the sperm, oocyte and early embryo.

Uterus

The uterus consists of the two uterine horns (cornua), and a small body (figure 11.2). Each horn is 2-3 feet in the non-pregnant sow. The uterine horns are long and tortuous that are freely movable because of the long broad ligaments. The degree to which the uterine horns are developed constitutes the basis of classification of the mammalian uteri. There are three distinct anatomical types of uteri namely (i) Duplex uterus (ii) bicornuate (iii) simplex

The Duplex uterus is characterized by two cervical canals that separate each uterine horn into distinct compartments. It is of two types.

- The first is characterized by having a single vaginal canal opening to the exterior. On the interior, it bifurcates (splits) into two vagina and two cervices. eg. Marsupials – Opossum- in this female will be inseminated by the male with a forked penis and deposits semen in each of the two sides of the reproductive tract simultaneously.

- In the second, less complex type of duplex uterus, there are two uterine horns with two distinct cervical canals connecting with a single vaginal canal. eg. rabbit. So it is possible to inseminate rabbit with two different male semen and obtain offsprings that will represent two different genetic types.

A Bicornuate uterus is characterized as having two uterine horns and a small uterine body. The length of the uterine horns is dependent on the degree of fusion between the paramesonephric ducts in the developing female fetus. In mare, where there is a high degree of fusion, there are short uterine horns and a relatively large uterine body. In cow, ewe and goat, there is a moderate degree of fusion resulting in uterine horns of intermediate length. In sow, very little fusion takes place between adjacent paramesonephric ducts resulting in long uterine horns. In all the types the uterus opens into the vagina through a single cervical canal.

The Simplex uterus is a fusion of the paramesonephric duct is almost complete, resulting in a single-chambered uterus without horns. eg. primates including humans.

Histology: The uterus consists of a thin outer layer, the perimetrium, thick myometrium composed of inner circular and outer longitudinal muscle layers and an inner layer, the endometrium. The outer perimetrium is the serous layer which is part of the peritoneum. In the myometrium, in between the inner circular and outer longitudinal layer of muscle fibres lies a vascular layer made of blood and lymph vessels, nerves and connective tissue. During pregnancy, the amount of muscle tissue in the uterine wall increases, both by cell enlargement and cell number.

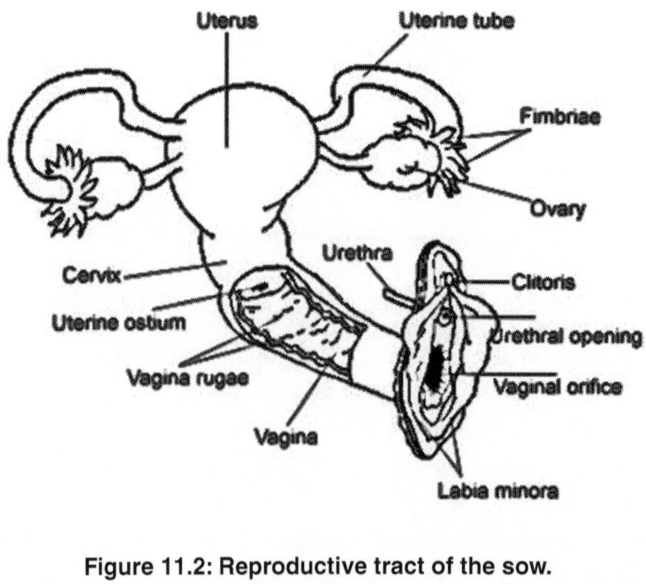

Figure 11.2: Reproductive tract of the sow.

The endometrium is a highly glandular structure consisting of an epithelial lining of the lumen, a glandular layer and connective tissue. The epithelial lining of the lumen is of a columnar cell type that undergoes structural change during pregnancy to facilitate the attachment of the blastocyst. The endometrium is characterized by numerous openings of the endometrial glands. These are simple branched tubular glands that are more or less coiled, especially towards their ends. The glands possess a lamellar connective tissue and are lined by simple or ciliated columnar epithelium. These glands are scattered throughout the endometrium with the exception of the caruncles. These uterine glands reach full secretary capacity under the influence of progesterone. These secretions called uterine milk or histrotroph are important to the survival and function of the preimplantation embryo. The function, thickness and vascularity of the structures of the endometrium are regulated by the changes in ovarian hormones throughout the estrous cycle and pregnancy.

Functions of the Uterus

- Sperm transport- The contraction of the myometrium is essential for the transport of spermatozoa from the site of ejaculation to the site of fertilization.
- Luteolysis and control of cyclicity- the uterus produces the PGF 2 that lysis the corpus luteum and thereby controls the oestrus cyclicity.
- Environment and pre-attachment embryo- uterus (endometrial glands) secrete the uterine milk which nourishes the free living zygote preceding implantation.
- Maternal contribution to the placenta- gives attachment to the placenta and plays a role in the nutrition, excretion and exchange of carbon dioxide and oxygen.
- Expulsion of the fetus and fetal placenta – at the time of parturition the strong muscular contractions of the uterus helps to expel the fetus and placenta.

Cervix

The cervix is a thick-walled, non-compliant organ between the vagina and uterus with a constricted lumen. It serves as a point of orientation during the clinical examinations of the genital organs. The canal of the cervix canalis cervices opens into the anterior vagina through the external os or os externum and into the uterus through the os uterinum or internal os. The cervical canal is characterized by various prominences. These prominences are in the form of transverse or spirally interlocking ridges known as annular rings. The rings are in a corkscrew arrangement that is adapted to the spiral twisting of the tip of the boar's penis. The junction of the cervix and vagina is a blind pouch called Fornix which is absent in sows.

Histology: Histologically the cervix consists of serosa, muscularis and mucosa. The mucosa is lined by tall columnar epithelial cells in between the goblet cells. During estrus, a thin stringy mucus is secreted while during pregnancy a thick tenacious mucus is secreted. The cervical wall is made up of fibroelastic collageneous tissue and muscular tissue. The collagen is responsible for the high tensile strength of the cervix.

The Function of the Cervix

- It prevents entry of pathogens into the uterus.
- Facilitates sperm transport.
- Acts as a sperm reservoir.
- Plays a vital role in the selection of viable sperms and prevents the transport of nonviable and defective sperms.
- Relaxes at the time of estrus and at the time of parturition to allow expulsion of the fetus.
- Increasing quantities of mucus is secreted at estrus and at pregnancy. During pregnancy the mucus thickens to form the cervical plug or seal.

Vagina

The vagina is the copulatory organ as well as the site for the expulsion of urine. It is a thin-walled structure, highly elastic and capable of considerable expansion. The vagina consists of serosa, muscular coat and mucosal layer. The mucosal epithelium varies depending on the region of the vagina. At the region near the cervix, the epithelium is columnar and highly secretory in nature. Towards the posterior vagina, the epithelium is of stratified squamous type, which thickens dramatically at the time of estrus. The bladder is connected to the vagina by the urethra.

Function of vagina

- Copulatory organ in which semen is deposited
- Acts as an excretory duct for the secretions of the cervix, uterus and oviduct.
- The cervical canal as well as the biochemical and microbiological milieu of the vagina protected the upper reproductive tract from invading microorganisms.

The Gartners ducts are blind sacs which are remnants of the Wolffian duct. Ventral to the urethral opening is the suburethral diverticulum in sow and cow. It is a blind pouch.

Vestibule

The vestibule in the sow is fairly long, about 7 to 9 cm. The labia are thick. The minor vestibular glands are variable in number. The clitoris is located about 2 cm cranial to the ventral commissure. On either side of the cranial portion of the floor of the vestibule, there is a cul-de-sac.

Vulva

The External part of the female reproductive tract. It often becomes red and swollen just prior to estrus and this swollen condition is usually more pronounced in gilts than in sows. The skin of the labia has numerous sebaceous and sweat glands. The labia consists of adipose tissue into which are embedded small bundles of smooth muscles which are called constrictor vulvae muscles.

11.2 Puberty and Sexual Maturity

Early attainment of age at puberty is important phenomenon for minimizing the cost associated with rearing and breeding replacement of gilts. Gilts that express estrus earlier after birth, can be mated at a time when they are physiologically more mature when compared to later developing gilts. These early puberty gilts produce more lifetime pigs per sow than gilts attain puberty late.

- Puberty is defined as the age or time at which the female or male gonads are able to produce gametes and reproduction may occur. In the female puberty is characterized by the appearance of estrum and ovulation. In males, it is characterized by secondary sexual changes and the ability to copulate and produce sperms.
- Sexual maturity is defined as the age or stage when an organism can reproduce, that means the production of fertile gametes (achievement of full sexual capacity in animals)
- Adolescence is the time of rapid changes in sexual development. In mid-adolescence both sexes become more interested in members of the opposite sex and seek heterosexual experience. The onset of puberty in swine is 5-8 months.

The mechanism of puberty is a complex process. It is associated with the maturation of the hypothalamic-pituitary axis. This axis is responsible for the release of hormones that must respond to positive hormonal feedback and also to the external stimuli. From birth to just prior to puberty, the hypothalamus is very sensitive to negative feedback inhibition of estrogen. During this time small amounts of estrogen are sufficient to inhibit gonadotropin synthesis and release. Under these conditions, follicles are not able to develop to a certain extent. At the time of puberty, two important events occur that establish ovarian cyclicity.

- There is a decrease in sensitivity of the hypothalamus to estrogen feedback- GnRH pulsatile release from the hypothalamus increases and gonadotropin secretion also increases. High frequency of GnRH pulses stimulates follicle development up to antrum formation and final follicle development.
- Secondly, increased secretion of estrogen results in positive feedback on the hypothalamus and anterior pituitary and gonadotrophin discharge. This gonadotrophin surge does not cause ovulation but causes significant production of progesterone form luteinized follicles. The progesterone

phase is short-lived and is followed in a few days by another surge of LH which leads to ovulation.

Factors affecting puberty

- Interaction with the opposite sex-Boar exposure
- Boar exposure has had the greatest impact on age at puberty in the gilt. It is clear that once-daily boar exposure induces estrus somewhat earlier. This effect is called as a boar effect. Particularly boars that are vocal can reduce the age at puberty compared to boars that do not utter any vocalization
- Influence of sex- female attains puberty at an earlier age
- Genetics-Fastest growing gilts expressed earlier puberty at a lighter weight.
- Climatic influence- animals in the tropics attain puberty at an early age
- Seasonal influence- Breeding season affects the onset of puberty. Eg. Gilts born in the spring and mature in the fall are delayed in pubertal age compared to gilts born in the fall and reach maturity in the spring
- Plane of nutrition- the high plane of nutrition leads to early puberty and undernourishment delays the onset of puberty. However, 20% of feed restrictions had no effect on the percentage of gilts expressing puberty.
- Bodyweight- gilts attain puberty after reaching a bodyweight of 64.9 to150.8kgs

❑❑❑

Chapter 12

Reproductive Physiology of Sows

—Dr. Berihu Gebrekidan & Dr. Gebregiorgis Ashebir

12.1 Estrus cycle and heat period

Oestrous cycle is the rhythmic sexual behavioral pattern developed in females after puberty. The combination of physiological events which begin with one estrous period and ends with the next is called oestrous cycle. The word `Oestrous' is derived from the Greek word `Oistros' meaning `Gad fly' –used to describe the behavior of cows when attacked by such flies. Based on the occurrence of oestrous cycles, animals are divided into:

- *Monoestrous:* animals showing only one estrous cycle per year e.g. Wild animals.
- *Polyestrous:* Animals exhibiting frequent, periodic estrous cycle per year e.g. cow and sow.
- *Seasonally polyestrous:* Animals exhibiting periodic estrous cycles only during a particular season e.g. Sheep and mare.

Depending on the ovarian activity again oestrous cycle is classified as

- *Regular oestrous cycle:* ovulation and formation of corpus luteum. Eg. Cow, sheep, mare, bitch and sow.
- *Spontaneous ovulators:* spontaneously ovulation will take place but CL formed will not be functional until mating has occurred e.g. rat or mouse.
- *Induced ovulators:* ovulation and CL formation depend on whether mating has occurred or not .e.g. cat, rabbit, mink.

Sows are non-seasonal and polyestrous and estrus is characterized by behavioral changes like mounting, fence walking, vocalizing, tilted ears and kyphosis and physical changes like vulvar swelling and vulval discharge

12.2 Stages of the estrous cycle

The estrous cycle is divided into two periods. Estrogenic or follicular phase comprising of proestrus and estrus and a progestational phase or luteal phase comprising of metestrus and diestrus.

Stages of estrus	*Duration*
Estrus	2 – 4 days
Metestrus	3-4 days
Diestrus	9 – 13 days
Proestrus	3 days

Proestrus

- Ill-defined period
- Growth of the Graafian follicle under the influence of FSH which results in increased production of estradiol 17
- Increased hyperplasia of myometrial cells
- Increased growth of cells and cilia of the oviduct
- Increased vascularity of uterine mucosa
- Increased thickness and vascularity of vaginal epithelium

Estrus

- Well defined period characterized by sexual desire and acceptance of male. The period begins with the first acceptance and ends with the last acceptance of the male
- Graafian follicle is large and mature
- Oviducts are tonic, epithelia mature and cilia are active, contractions of oviduct occur, the fimbriated end of the oviduct assumes close affinity to the Graafian follicle. Increased amounts of oviductal fluid secreted
- Uterus is erect and turgid. Increased blood supply and increased growth of mucosa. Mucous is secreted.
- Vaginal mucosa pink and congested due to increased vascularity
- Thickening of vaginal mucosa in dogs and cats. Increased desquamation of cornified epithelial cells
- Cervix relaxed and oedematous
- Stringy mucous hangs from the vulva
- Increased neutrophilic infiltration into the uterine lumen

In most species, ovulation takes place during oestrus but in cows, ovulation occurs 12 hours after the end of estrus. In induced ovulators such as rabbit and mink, ovulation does not take place until mating occurs. In cat, estrum may be prolonged in the absence of a male to 7 to 10 days.

Metestrum

- Transitional period between ovulation and full development of corpus luteum
- Poorly defined period
- Largely under influence of progesterone produced by the CL. Inhibits FSH secretion and prevents the development of more Graafian follicles
- In cows, growth of endometrial glands begins, capillary hemorrhage occurs and post estrual bleeding or metestrual bleeding due to withdrawal of estrogen takes place
- In primates, loss of superficial layers of endometrium called as mensuration takes place due to the withdrawal of progesterone
- Decreased mucus secretion
- Uterus becomes less tonic
- In queens not bred, no ovulation and CL formation. The follicles become atretic.

Diestrum

- Longest phase or period of the cycle
- CL matures. There is a progesterone effect on the uterus takes place. There is increased hypertrophy of the endometrial gland, and increased thickening of the endometrium
- Cervix closed and vaginal mucous scanty
- Vaginal mucous membrane pale
- Uterine muscles are flaccid.

12.3 Endocrine Control of Oestrous Cycle

The Oestrous cycle consists of two phases –the follicular phase and the luteal phase. The follicular phase of oestrous cycle is initiated and regulated by the release of GnRH from the two centers, tonic and surge centers of the hypothalamus. The Ventromedial nucleus and arcuate nucleus of the hypothalamus form the tonic GnRH center, which is responsible for the basal secretion of GnRH in small pulses over a substantial period of time.

The CNS receives information from the environment of the animal and conveys this information to the hypothalamus. Within the hypothalamus endocrine neurons release GnRH. This GnRH is transported via the hypothalamo hypophyseal portal system and reaches the anterior pituitary where it stimulates the synthesis and secretion of LH and FSH from anterior pituitary gonadotrophs.

Early stages of follicular development are independent of gonadotrophin support. However, FSH and LH are required for antrum formation and for development beyond 4 mm diameter. The dynamics of antral follicles involves three major events, recruitment, selection and dominance.

- High levels of FSH, low concentration of LH and no inhibin initiates follicular recruitment from a pool of ovarian follicles
- Selection of healthy follicles is achieved by moderate levels of FSH, LH and low levels of inhibin.
- The dominant or ovulatory follicle is characterized by low levels of FSH, high levels of LH and inhibin

Within the selected follicles, LH binds with LH receptors located on the theca interna of the developing follicles and activates the conversion of cholesterol to testosterone. Testosterone then diffuses into granulosa cells and gets aromatized to estradiol 17 beta under the influence of FSH. Two cells, theca and granulosa cells and two hormones, FSH and LH are involved in the production of estrogen. Hence called as two cell Two Gonadotropin theory.

- As the selected follicles continue to grow to the dominant stage it causes suppression of other follicles larger than 4 mm diameter. Estrogen and inhibin secretions increase. The increased concentration of inhibin exhibits negative feedback on FSH release from the anterior pituitary resulting in atresia of unselected follicles.
- As estrogen levels reach a threshold, it stimulates the surge center namely the preoptic and suprachiasmatic nucleus of the hypothalamus and causes GnRH surge which in turn stimulates LH surge leading to ovulation.

After ovulation, the theca interna and the granulosa cells of the follicle undergo luteinization, a process governed by LH. Immediately after ovulation the walls of the follicle collapse into many folds. These folds begin to interdigitate, allowing thecal cells and granulosa cells to mix. The luteal tissue consists of large and small luteal cells. The large cells originate from granulosa cells and secrete oxytocin and progesterone. The small cells originate from cells of theca interna and secrete progesterone.

The progesterone stimulates hypertrophy of endometrial glands, increases uterine milk secretions, inhibits contractions of the uterus and prevents neutrophilic infiltration. Progesterone also plays an important role in the endocrine control of reproduction because it exerts strong negative feedback on the hypothalamus thereby preventing the development of preovulatory follicles (follicles develop during luteal phase but do not reach preovulatory stage unless progesterone decreases), production of estrogen, behavioraloestrus, preovulatory surge of GnRH and LH.

If the animal is not pregnant, the CL undergoes luteolysis. Luteal oxytocin and PGF2 alpha from endometrium cause luteolysis. Estrogen from the follicular waves cause formation of oxytocin receptors in the uterus. The oxytocin from the CL binds to oxytocin receptors in the endometrium and activates the enzyme system necessary for formation of PGF2 alpha. The PGF2 alpha reaches the ovaries by a vascular countercurrent exchange system.

Luteolysis is brought about by:

- Reduction in blood flow to the CL by vasoconstriction

- PGF2 alpha binds to specific receptors on large luteal cells causing influx of Ca ions. High intracellular Ca ions is thought to cause apoptotic effects (programmed cell death)
- PGF2 alpha receptor complex also activates protein kinase C (PK-C) which inhibits progesterone synthesis

The lysis of CL results in decreased progesterone levels. The negative block on hypothalamus is removed and a new cycle is initiated.

12.4 Factors Affecting Estrous Cycle

- *Nutrition:* Inanition or starvation caused by lack of energy or nutritional deficiency impairs or prevents secretions of gonadotropic hormones from pituitary gland.
- *Temperature:* Excessive heat during summer months causes decreased thyroid activity which directly reduces reproductive efficiency.
- *Age:* In swine the young female usually has a slightly shorter length of estrous cycle than the adult animals. Similarly causes cessation of estrous cycle.
- *Systemic diseases:* Severe chronic wasting diseases cause debility and emaciation resulting in cessation of estrous cycle.
- *Pathology of uterus and cervix:* Conditions like pyometra, fetal maceration, mummification causes persistence of corpus luteum and cessation of estrous cycle.
- *Endocrine disturbances:* Endocrine disturbances leading to cystic ovaries or pituitary, ovarian and adrenal tumors affect the length of the oestrous cycle.
- *Miscellaneous causes:* Pregnancy causes physiological cessation of estrous cycle. The presence of males hastens onset of estrous. Infusion of iodine compounds into the uterus shortens the oestrous cycle.

12.5 Heat Detection

Common signs of heat

- When the reproductive efficiency of a herd depends on proper heat detection and correct time of insemination, it is important for one to know what signs to look for and when to look for them.
- Females of every species exhibit estrus signs for a certain amount of time during their estrous cycle. While most of these signs are similar among species, there are some that are species specific.
- Signs that signal the onset of estrus can be classified as primary or secondary. Primary signs are most reliable while secondary signs are less reliable as they vary in length and intensity and may be confused with the symptoms that are indicators of minor health problems such as increased urination, isolation and decreased feed intake.

- The best time to observe for signs of estrus are during the coolest times of the day, early in the morning, before feeding and milking, early afternoon and late evening, after the animals have finished eating and before or after milking.
- Immobilization
- Redness and swelling of the vulva, increase in vaginal secretions
- Off feed, rooting or mounting penmates
- Nudging other females
- Vocalization
- Erect or "perked" ears
- Moist vulva
- Desire to seek out boars
- moist vulva

Detection of heat: Successful swine breeding and high conception rate depends on the ability to identify the sow or gilt in heat

- Vulval swelling, reddening of vulva is noticed 2-6 days prior to oestrus. reddening are readily detectable in gilts but more difficult to identify in case of sows
- In some case vaginal discharge is noticed (figure 12.1)

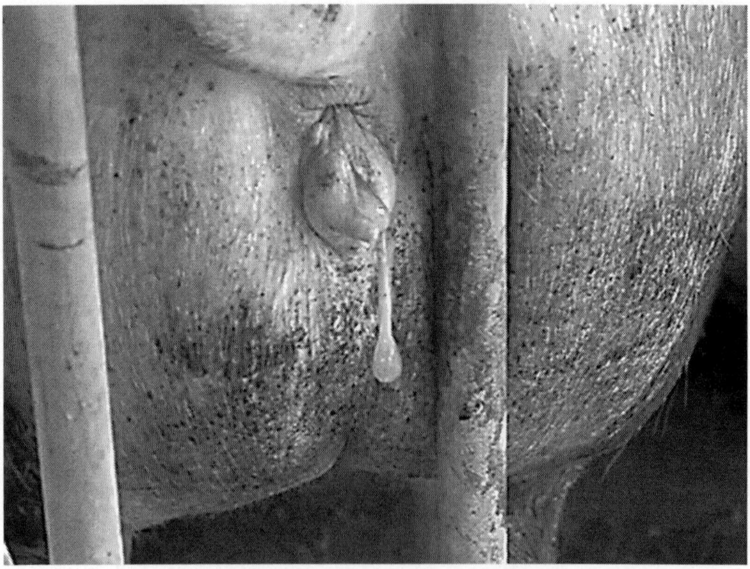

Figure 12.1: Vaginal discharge with swollen vulva.

- The animal will be restless and the activity level will be increased and a typical grunt indicates pig in heat

- Oestrus gilts frequently mount on other sows and allow them to be mounted
- 'Standing heat reflex' will be exhibited during oestrus. Which describes the female mating stance and this consist of immobilization, arching back and in some breed cocking of ears are noticed.

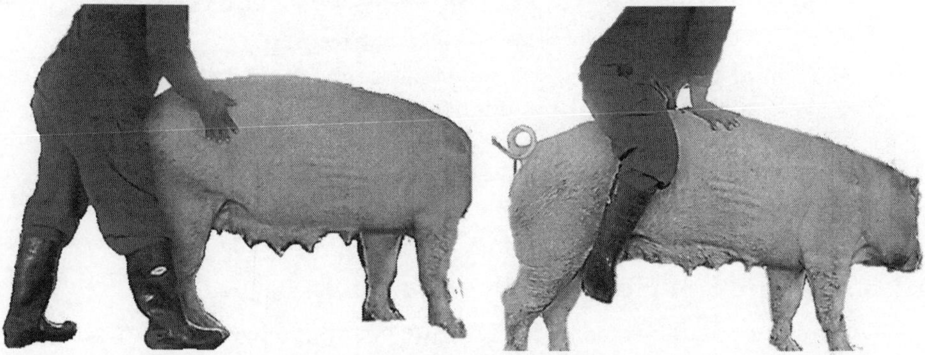

Figure 12.2: Standing heat reflex and riding test for heat detection

- Another important symptom which known as standing heat test or riding test or back pressure test in is the sow remains immobile with erected ear when normal pressure is applied to lumbo-sacral region (figure 12.2). This test can be performed in front of boar or adjacent to a boar pen. This method is the ideal method for heat detection in pigs.
- Reduced appetite, frequent urination, mounting and standing for mounting can also be considered as heat symptoms.

Estrus Detection Aids

- Detection aids are needed in most herds in order to overcome the difficulty of estrus detection so that all animals in estrus are effectively identified and bred either naturally or artificially.
- In addition to the use of accurate record systems and induced ovulation programmes, there are a variety Estrus of additional aids to estrus detection. Traditional methods include pressure sensitive mount detectors, tail head markings, and detector animals. Newer concepts include monitoring of electrical resistance of reproductive tract tissue, pedometry and electronic pressure-sensitive mount detectors.
- However, it should be borne in mind that these are only aids and should be used only in conjunction with visual detection programmes and not as a substitute for visual detection.
- Heat detection in sows can be done by performing a back pressure test where the herds person applies pressure on the back flanks and underline of the sow simulating the action or feeling of a boar mounting a sow. If the sow stands rigid and "locks up" in expectation of being mounted and bred by a boar, then she is in estrus. An attempt to run away during

application of back pressure indicates that she is not in estrus. Along with the immobile stance "cocking" of the ears or twitching if she is a floppy –eared breed indicates that the sow is in estrus.

- Pedometers: Pedometers to measure the increased activity around estrus have been successfully used to detect estrus in sows. Recently, with the development of miniaturized accelerometers and infrared sensors, the efficiency of heat detections has increased.
- Vaginal Electrical Resistance: Measurement of the vaginal electrical resistance or vaginal impedance appears to be a useful method for objectively determining the occurrence of estrus. However, the problems associated with the use of these methods were the large fluctuations due to the depth of the probe in the vagina and the pressure of the hand while carrying out the measurement.

12.6 Induction of Heat in Gilts and Sows

Five minutes of daily contact with mature boar is sufficient to stimulate early puberty in gilts providing gilts have adequate opportunity for both physical and visual contact with the boars. Gilts that are of 165 days of age appear to require daily boar exposure to obtain rapid and maximum pubertal response. Similarly serum gonadotropin treatment will also induce heat in 3 - 5 days. In case of sows weaning of litter itself will induce oestrus.

12.7 Mating Methods

Hand mating: In this method bring the sows to the boar for individual service when they are in standing heat. It most common method of mating in pure bred herds. In this method the boar is more efficiently used. The farrowing rate is more accurate. The repeat breeder and sterile sows can be detected easily and culled regularly. Breeding defects can be detected easily.

Pen mating: in this method one boar is allowed in the sow pen (8-10) for detecting heat and mating. There is a chance for over usage of boar. Record maintenance in this method is difficult.

Flock or herd mating: in this method the boar is permitted for run with the sows. Mature boar can usually satisfactorily serve 15-20 sows in pasture mating system. Young boars not more than 8 to 10 gilts.

12.8 Mating Management

- After detecting heat the sow and boar should be introduced in a familiar area so as to facilitate better mating.
- Young boar must be handled carefully. Hand mating is good in young boar. It is better to use young boar to experienced sow and experienced adult boar to gilts
- If new boar is introduced in to the herd, he should not be used until after a minimum period of 30 days of isolation.

- Boars not familiar with each other should be kept together since it may result in fatal fighting.
- The fertility of the boar should be tested at least 30 days before using him in a herd. One of the best ways is to mate him to five or six healthy gilt that is to be marketed. If more than one gilt return to heat in 28 days after mating, the fertility of the boar will be questionable
- A yearling boar can serve 10 to 15 female and can be expected to serve 7 to 8 gilt per week
- When temperature exceeds 27 C hand mating should be done early in the morning or late in the evening
- The sow should be bred at least twice preferably during late hours on the first day and early hours on the second day which will increase the conception rate by 30% in first heat and increase the litter size by one
- Sometimes boars may be aggressive and cause physical trauma to the female. Hence experienced stock should be familiar with any variation to be expected to prevent problems arising.
- Prompt recording of mating process should be done which facilitate the recording of mating, boar performance and sow performance. This will help in future culling of poor performing sows and boars.
- Patience and good judgment is necessary in handling the breeding animals. Rough treatment may cause old boar to become vicious or young boar to become reluctant and they may not mate readily when needed.
- Sow ovulate 16-48 hours after the onset of estrous and it will lose its fertility rate rapidly, hence it is better to breeding during the latter half of the first day or early on the second day of estrous
- Sometime gilt may show standing heat symptom on the next day and that animal should be re-mated with 12-14 hour interval
- Sow normally come to heat one to four days after farrowing but it is better to mate during the first heat after weaning the litter
- Ovulation rate increases during successive estrous [up to fifth] thus it is advantageous to delay breeding of gilts until the second or third estrous

12.9 Ovulation

Ovulation is the release of oocyte from mature Graafian follicle. Ovulation in mammalian ovary occurs on any point in the ovarian surface.

Theories of ovulation:

1. *Follicular pressure theory:* As the follicle grows the amount of liquor folliculi also increases. This liquor folliculi exerts pressure on the follicular wall thereby follicles rupture. However, this was not the case with cystic ovaries where there was both an increase in follicular size and follicular fluid but there was no rupture. Theory not accepted.

2. *High osmotic pressure theory:* Liquor folliculi consists of more amount of electrolytes particularly Na and K. Increased osmotic pressure leads to rupture of the follicle. In cystic ovaries size of the follicle and amount of follicular fluids along with electrolyte content also increased but still there was no rupture. Hence, theory was disagreed.
3. *Ischemic theory:* Increased follicular fluid exerts pressure against follicular wall. At one point due to pressure, ischemia occurs and leads to stigma formation and ovulation. Theory partly accepted.
4. *Follicular wall thinning and rupture:* Nearing ovulation, the blood supply to the follicle increases Thinning of the follicular wall occurs at one point called as stigma. Ovarian contractions and follicular rupture occurs. Theory accepted.

Recent theory is that ovulation is a combination of physiological, biochemical and biophysical mechanisms.

A Surge of LH occurs at the beginning of oestrus prior to ovulation when progesterone is at its minimal levels and oestradiol has reached its highest cyclical values. Several tissue layers separate the oocyte from the outside of the follicle. These are the surface epithelium, the tunica albugenia, theca externa, and interna, basement membrane and granulosa cells. All these tissue layers have to be broken down before ovulation can take place.

An increased blood flow near ovulation occurs to all classes of follicles but the follicle destined to ovulate receives the largest volume of blood and has capillaries more permeable then those in other follicle. As the follicle enlarges it begins to protrude from the surface of the ovaries, the vascularity of the follicular surface increases except at its center, which is devoid of blood vessels. This avascular area is the future point of rupture. Meanwhile there is dissociation of cumulus cells which detaches the oocyte from the membrana granulosa and now the oocyte is surrounded by the radiata cells. Resumption of Meiosis (Nuclear Maturation) occurs 3 hours after LH surge and ends 1 hour before ovulation when the first polar body is extruded. Cumulus cells actively secrete a viscous mass enclosing the oocyte and its corona. After follicular rupture the viscous mass spreads at the ovarian surface to facilitate the pickup of oocytes by the fimbriae.

The LH surge also causes a temporary shift in steroid secretions by increasing progesterone secretion. This progesterone stimulates collagenase activity in the follicular wall reading to dissociation of bundles of collagen fibers (increase in plasmin activity causes an increase in follicular wall elasticity). The LH surge also causes an increase of PGF2 and PGE2 levels. These prostaglandins play a basic role in follicular rupture, and inhibition of their synthesis prevents ovulation. PGE2 stimulates production of plasminogen activator thus increasing plasmin activity which increase in follicular wall elasticity and is involved in tissues cell migration and thereby causes mixing of theca and granulosa cells during CL formation.

PGF2α causes rupture of the epithelial cell lysosomes at the follicular epithelium. Their hydrolase's destroy the underlying albugenia cells and then the theca cells.

After lysosomal rupture, epithelial cells scale off. The wall of the follicular apex becomes thin in a circumscribed area called the stigma. The PGF2 causes contraction of the smooth muscle cells that are present in the ovarian stroma and theca externa thus leading to ovarian contractions Ovulation and follicular contractions. These ovarian contractions cause follicular rupture and follicular contractions causes expulsion of the oocyte.

At the time of ovulation the ovum, together with surrounding cells in a gelatinous mass, protrudes at the ovarian surface and is swept into the ostium of the oviduct by the action of the motile kinocilia of the fimbriae.

Ovulation occurs in most gilts during the latter part of the second day after the onset of estrus however the time between the onset of estrus and ovulation varies considerably.

12.10 Gestation

Care and management of sows during gestation

Record the date of mating to determine the expected date of farrowing. Pregnancy can be detected either by visual inspection or by means of an ultrasound device. Keep sty clean, dry, non-slippery and provide 2.7m 2 per animal. Do not allow to mix pregnant gilts/ sows with other animals to avoid fighting which may lead to skidding. Provide an adequate physical environment for bred females to avoid stress. Provide bedding 8 - 10 cm chopped straw under covered area. Allow the animal for grazing to leguminous greens. Feed bred females a 16 % protein ration at a rate of 2.0 to 2.5 kg per day for first 75 days after breeding. Do not over feed, increase the feeding level to 3 to 3.5 kg per day last 35 to 45 days of gestation.

Gestational weight gain should be 25 to 35 kg. Vaccinate bred sows/gilts for infectious disease of swine, 20 to 30 days before farrowing. Deworming gilts and sows 3 to 4 weeks before expected date of farrowing. Control external parasites, particularly lice and mange infestation give medicated wallow only after they have been watered. Keep plenty of clean water available at all times. Provide sufficient exercise to the pregnant sows during the gestation period usually have less difficulty at farrowing and they often produce pigs which are more vigorous than those produced by sows which have not had ample exercise.

12.11 Pregnancy Diagnosis

Accurate means of diagnosing pregnancy is an essential part of any commercial breeding programme. Early detection of non-pregnancy would

- Provide a means of identifying and combating fertility problems in groups or individuals at as early a stage as possible.
- Assists the economy and efficiency of flock or herd management by identifying non-pregnant animals which can be culled or served again
- Help in certification of pregnancy in individual animals which will be important for both selling and buying.

Thus, an accurate method of determining pregnancy/ non-pregnancy before the expected second estrus would be ideal.

Signs of pregnancy

- Female become more docile during pregnancy and the physical activity will be reduced due to increase in weight during advanced pregnancy
- The development of mammary system is another indication of pregnancy. Secretions in the lumen of the duct begin by 75th day of pregnancy and by 90th day the enlargement of gland is easily visible. By about 114 days [a few hours before parturition] the glands are full of colostrum and lactation begins when the first piglet is born. Normally gilts will show some signs of udder development after 2 months of pregnancy. A sow normally shows signs of new udder development some 2 to 3 weeks before farrowing.
- Sometime pregnant sow may show signs of excitement and often bite walls and fences seeking outlet
- 1 to 3 days before farrowing the pitch of voice may be lowered and the sow may begin to prepare nest for her litter
- Farrowing in the morning and early afternoon is a rare thing, normally farrowing appears to follow a diurnal pattern, more frequently in late afternoon and most frequently at night
- Duration of farrowing varies from 2 to 24 hours in normal parturition. The sow often takes rest in between expulsion of piglets.

Pregnancy diagnosis

Traditionally, failure to return to estrus at 18-22 days after service or artificial insemination has been regarded as a sign of pregnancy. However, the detection of estrus can be difficult due to a reluctance to show signs, anoestrus or ovarian cysts, and is time-consuming and inconsistent. It is important to know as soon as possible if a sow or gilt is not pregnant so that she can be served again, treated or culled. A reliable method is also necessary so that breeders can certify that an animal is pregnant before sale. Any technique must be accurate, capable of being used early in gestation and fairly inexpensive.

Rectal palpation

Rectal palpation depends upon palpation per rectum of the cervix, uterus and middle uterine arteries.

0-21 Days

- The cervix and uterus feel very similar to their state at diestrus
- During this period the bifurcation of the cornua becomes less distinct and the uterus becomes slightly enlarged, with soft walls.
- The middle uterine artery increases to approximately 5 mm in diameter towards the third week.

1-30 Days

- The bifurcation of the cornua is less distinct, the cervix and uterine walls are flaccid and thin.
- The middle uterine artery is 5-8 mm in diameter and more easily identified.

31-60 Days

- The cervix feels like a soft-walled tubular structure
- The uterus is ill defined and thin walled.
- The middle uterine artery is enlarged to about the same size as the external iliac artery.
- Fremitus can be first identified at 35 to 37 days and the pulse pattern can be compared with that of the external iliac artery.

60 days to term

- The middle uterine artery is greater in diameter than the external iliac and it has strong fremitus; it now crosses the external iliac artery more dorsally than before.
- Only towards the end of gestation is it possible to palpate piglets at the level of the cornual bifurcation. The technique can be performed without the need of much restraint, preferably when the animal is feeding. Unfortunately, it is not possible to perform the technique in gilts because they are too small, and even in large sows a slender arm is advantageous.

Ultrasonic methods

B-mode direct imaging has proved to be very successful in the sow. The transducer probe is applied to the abdominal wall of the standing sow about 5 cm posterior to the umbilicus, to the right of the umbilicus and is directed towards the posterior abdomen. Errors may be due to prenatal death.

Vaginal biopsy

Histological assessment of the number of layers of the stratified squamous epithelium of the vaginal mucosa obtained by biopsy can be used as a method of diagnosing pregnancy in the sow. The accuracy of this method between 30 and 90 days after service is 97 and 94% for the diagnosis of pregnancy and non-pregnancy respectively. The diagnosis depends on the number of layers of vaginal epithelial cells, which in turn, relates to the endocrine state: thus during pro-estrus, when estrogen is dominant, a rapid proliferation of the stratum germinatum occurs so that at estrus there are up to 20 layers. From the end of estrus and throughout the luteal phase, when progesterone is dominant, the depth of vaginal epithelium falls so that by day 11 or 12 there are only three or four irregularly arranged layers and only two or three layers in late diestrus. With the onset of pregnancy, progesterone domination continues, and by day 26, the typical histological picture is two parallel rows of epithelial cells with condensed darkly staining nuclei. The best time to test is from 18 to 25 days after mating.

Sections taken erroneously from the cervix or posterior vagina are unsatisfactory for diagnosis. False-negative results are probably due to errors in the processing of the tissue or mistaken identification of the animal or sample. Disadvantages are cost of the procedure and delay in knowing the results.

Estimation of Plasma Progesterone

Sows bled 16-24 days after service and subjected to plasma progesterone estimations were diagnosed as pregnant when values in plasma were > 7.5 ng/ ml. Accuracy of the test was 96 % and because of irregularities of the interestrus interval, the test was more reliable in identifying those sows non pregnant. The disadvantage was the difficulty in obtaining samples.

Plasma Estrogen Assay

Estrone sulphate in the blood of pregnant animals can be detected from day 20 of gestation and therefore can be used as a method for diagnosing pregnancy. Maximum concentrations are present around days 24-28.

12.12 Artificial insemination

Artificial insemination (AI) is a process by which sperms are collected from the male, processed, stored and artificially introduced into the female reproductive tract of the same species for the purpose of conception. In short AI is the introduction of semen into the vagina of a female by same means other than sexual intercourse. It is an important technique for improving the genetic quality of domesticated animals. It has been widely used in swine throughout the world.

- *Benefits:* The genetic influence of superior boars can be spread widely.
- *Increase uniformity:*AI makes development of large number of animals with a superior family possible, they providing uniformity and better bases for a constructive breeding and sale program.
- *Economical service:* Cost of maintenance of boar is reduced (only fewer sires required - 1:150 boar- to sow ratio routinely achieved).
- *Better health program:* AI stops venereal contact reproductive problems in individual females one more easily detected and the fertility of the males can be detected at an early age.
- *Improved herd records:* Sire and breeding dates of each offspring are known and more accurate herd records are observation results in improved culling and management.
- *Safety:* Not having a male animal on the premises eliminates the potential danger of aggressive males that could cause harm to the producer.
- *Rapid proof for sire:* Progeny testing examination on the offspring of the particular boar within a short time for desired traits with natural mating wood only have 100's of offspring only.

- *Availability:* Sires are available anywhere in the world. Even after death of the male, semen can be used. Oldest frozen semen 40-45 years old. Old and crippled boars are also used for AI by collecting semen through electro ejaculation/rectal massage.
- *Shorten duration:* Produce genetically superior i.e. fast growing with lean meat sows in a shorter duration.
- *Accessibility:* Easier access for consumers to obtaining high quality semen.
- Elimination of infertile animal:Early detection of infertile boars and eliminate it from the breeding program.
- *Limitation of AI:* Reduced farrowing rate(50%) with frozen semen
- *Storing time:* Lower than average results with chilled semen stored longer than 72 hours.
- *Human detection of heat:* a very detailed management practices is required because success or failures depends on how well heat is detected in the female population.
- *Required a skilled technical:* Proper training and experience and patience are essential to be successful with AI.
- *Maybe subject of abuses:* Because it is impossible to differentiate between the semen of individuals of the same species, the integrity technicians and semen collection agencies is very important.
- *May accentuate the damage:* From the poor boar: because a greater number of offspring is available through AI, an inferior sire can increase his negative influence.
- *Requires additional capital and management:* Due to extra labor and facilities which are usually required because of extra handling for insemination of each individual.
- *Species variation:* Boar semen is not that much good when compared to bull semen for frozen semen storage.
- *Storage:* Technology to store cooled or frozen semen is difficult

The following are the insemination techniques for chilled and frozen semen deposition. Insemination can be done by any one of the following methods.

Chilled or liquid semen

Equipment

- Semen: Liquid semen-Keep the semen in the storage container until use
    - Frozen semen - In liquid nitrogen container until use.
- Scissors- to cut the twist-off caps/frozen semen straws
- Towel or damp paper
- Disposable insemination rods
- Sex odour Aerosol or mature boar in the adjacent pen
- Non-spermicidal jelly for lubrication.
- Oxytocin, a syringe and needle.

Insemination Technique

- Make sure that the sow is in standing heat. To confirm the standing heat, look for ear popping, sticky mucous and an engorged clitoris in addition to the standing heat.
- Clean the vulva with a damp paper or towel.
- To stimulate uterine contractions allow nose to nose contact with a mature boar in the adjacent pen. Rub the animal flanks and put some weight on her back before and during insemination
- Two minutes before artificial insemination oxytocin injection can be given to stimulate uterine contraction that aids semen intake. This may improve conception rates and litter size.
- Two common styles of rods are present in the market
    - Spirette-type insemination rods. It is counter clockwise threads on the tip.
    - Rods with a rounded foam tip

While using a spirette type insemination rod, the tip is lubricated with extender or little lubricating jelly. The rod is gently inserting into the vulva. While passing the rod into the vulva it should be gently guided with the tip pointing up through the vagina to the cervix. To avoid the entry of rod into the bladder. Gently twist the rod counter clockwise as it is being inserted. After passing 8-10 inches, pus the rod gently and continue to twist counter clockwise until the tip is locked in to the cervix. Ascertain whether the tip of the rod is locked into the cervix

The foam tipped rods or squeeze and please rods are inserted like threaded rods, but do not need to be rotated. Slowly push the rod until you feel the foam tip catch in the folds of the cervix. Test the lock by pulling back gently on the rod.

Insemination: Remove the tip of the semen container and insert it into the end of the rod. If need apply gentle pressure to the bottle. Do not force the semen into the animal. Gentle squeezing favours the semen to flow into the animal. It may take 5 minutes or more to complete the bottle. Continue to stimulate the animal by putting weight on her back and rubbing her flanks. A bit of semen backflow at the vulva is normal. Reposition the rod tip if much back flow of semen is seen. After emptying the semen bottle remove it from rod and draw some air into the bottle and reattached into the bottle. Gently use the air to force the last quantity of semen from the rod. Then rotate the rod clockwise and withdraw it.

Insemination with foam tipped rod: Inside the rod is a rubber sleeve that is attached to the tip. During insemination, hydraulic pressure turns the sleeve inside out and the sleeve threads through the cervix and deposits semen directly into the uterus. After positioning the rod, wait two to three minutes for attachment of the semen bottles. Forcefully squeeze the bottle after attachment. You will feel the pressure release when the sleeve is completely inverted. When the sleeve is inverted, remove the bottle from the rod, draw a small quantity of air into the bottle and reattach. This force any remaining semen out of the rod. Actual insemination takes only a few seconds. 12 to 24 hours after insemination check the animal for standing heat. If the sow is in standing heat even after 24 hours after artificial insemination re inseminate the sow with second dose of semen.

Measures to ensure that maximum numbers of bred pigs settle and farrow large litters or management for optimal production

The fertility of sow and litter size farrowed and weaned are very important factors in determining the viability of swine projects. The cost of raising 6 pigs or 10 pigs from birth to weaning is more or less similar since the maintenance requirement of the sows is the same to both cases. Breeding and selection alone are not very certain methods of improving the production of swine. Time spent on improving the management of the sow and litter, on increasing the efficiency of feed utilization and the control of diseases are parasites may contribute more to the income of the enterprise than an equal time spent to increase herd productivity by following complex method of breeding and selection.

To ensure that the maximum number of bred gilts and sows farrow large litter of living pigs the following measures are suggested.

- Gilt may be bred to farrow at 12-14 months of age. Gilts should weigh at least 100 kg before breeding.
- Gilts come into heat during first few days after weaning. When weaned after 3 weeks breed on the first heat.
- In hand breeding sows are bred twice during the heat period. Once when they come into heat and again after 24 hours. In pen mating sow may be put with a boar till the heat lasts.
- The commercial pig may be bred to several boars in the same heat period. 2 boars are run together with the same female in heat or 1 boar for 1 day and second for next. With this procedure the chance of conception will increase.
- Though the heritability of litter size is low. Selecting for this trait should be continued. In order to increase the litter size by 1 pig we may have to select pigs for this trait for 20 generations.
- The female selected for breeding must haveat least 12 functional and well-spaced teatsand a good body length.
- While selecting the breed for a swine enterprise the litter size must be kept in mind. Yorkshire pigs are on the top in this regard with 10-11 pigs per litter. In most breeds litter size is 9-10 but in few breeds it may be as low as 6-8.
- If old boars are to be used for breeding, one with a good conception rate with large litters may be used.
- Both the gilts and sows must be thrifty and in medium condition before breeding, of too fat, the condition may be reduced and if too thin, the condition may be improved.
- During hot summer months one must keep the breeding and gestating sows cool by water sprinkling or by the use of wallow.

- Intense inbreeding may be avoided as for each 10% inbreeding there is one-third less pig per litter farrowed and one-half pig less at weaning.
- Before breeding check the females for brucellosis and leptospirosis. One must avoid breeding sows suffering from flu. During early gestation high body temperature at breeding time may cause abortion.
- Gilts and sows may be kept in the farrowing stall or pen 5-7 days before due to farrow.
- A well trained attendant is needed for farrowing. As soon as newborn pigs are dried after removing membranes, it is made sure they breathe. Overlying should be prevented. Greatest losses occur within 3 days after farrowing, so a close watch on the sows and pigs must be maintained during that period. The death may be due to starvation (26%), digestive problem (2%) and unknown cause (13%).
- The sow is at her best in milk production at about 3 weeks lactation after which milk quantity is reduced. So a creep feed may be used from 3 weeks till weaning to supplement milk. The ideal weaning weight at 8 weeks age is 15 kg.
- The farrowing and nursing facilities between groups of females farrowed must be cleaned and kept vacant for at least a week.
- The sow and pigs must be put on 'clean pasture'. More than 6 sow and litter per lot may not be put on the pasture.

General guide line for normal reproduction of pigs

Age at puberty	6-7 months
Breeding age of gilts	8 -9 months
Breeding weight of gilts	80-90 kg
Breeding age of boar	1 - 1 ½ years
Sex ratio	1:10
Estrus cycle	19-23 days average 21 days
Estrus period	2-3 days
Mating time	Gilt first day and sow second day of onset of heat
Time of ovulation	16 – 48 hours after onset of oestrus
Number of service per conception	Two at an interval of 12-24 hours
Gestation period	114 days (3 months, 3 weeks, 3 days)
Suckling period	56 days
Average litter size at birth	10-12
Average litter weight at birth	12-14 kg
Birth weight	1.2-1.3 kg
Average litter size at weaning	8-10
Average litter weight at weaning	120 kg in gilts and 150 kg in sows
Weaning weight	12-13 kg

Occurrence of heat after weaning	4-7 days
Volume of ejaculate	200 ml
Average number of sperms per ml	100,000
Average age to castrate pigs	2-3 weeks
Market age of fattening pigs	5 and 7th months
Market weight at 6 months	70-75 kg in Indian condition
Farrowing interval	7-7 ½ months
Farrowing rate	1.8-1.9
Average life of sow	6 litters

❑❑❑

Chapter 13

Selection of Swine

— Dr. Berihu Gebrekidan

Selection of pig can be done for many purpose. Pigs can be selected for slaughtering purpose where they are kept for few days in farm or sent immediately for slaughtering to earn money in short span of time. Selection of feeder pigs are done at early stage and they were fed until they attain market weight. Then they are sold as slaughtering pig to the trader or directly sent for slaughter. The primary reason for selecting breeding stock is to genetically upgrade your herd. Proper animal selection is one foundation of successful swine production. The choices made will affect producers' profits far into the future. Selection is important in many ways, from producing quality pork to animal health.

The swine population is large and consists of several breeds. Personal preference and/or individual merit of the hog are the basis for the selection of a breed. No one breed is perfect in every respect. Breeds of swine are commonly chosen by producers to meet the conditions under which the hogs are to be raised. The producers need to establish why they are raising hogs; for breeding stock or to sell at the market. Individual merits of the animal are the key to establishing and maintaining a profitable herd, particularly if the objective is to produce and sell breeding stock. Today, a structurally sound, healthy, thick muscled, highly efficient hog with a large body capacity is considered the "ideal" hog. Highly controlled selection and breeding programs within breeds and specialized crossbreeding programs have put the swine industry near the top in production among the various livestock enterprises.

Breeds of swine can be grouped into two different categories, maternal and terminal breeds. The maternal breeds are known for their large litters and are selected for replacement females. Terminal sire breeds are recognized for their growth and carcass quality and are usually used for terminal crosses. Chester White, Landrace and Yorkshire are the most common maternal breed while Berkshire, Duroc,

Hampshire, Spot, Poland China, Pietrain are some of the important terminal sire breeds.

13.1 Selection of Slaughter and Feeder Pig

Differentiation between slaughter and feeder swine is based solely on their intended use rather than on specific identifiable characteristics of the swine. Slaughter swine are those which are intended for slaughter immediately or in the near future. Feeder swine are those which are intended for slaughter after a period of feeding. The grade of a feeder pig is determined by evaluating two general value-determining characteristics. That is its logical slaughter potential and its thriftiness. The logical slaughter potential of a thrifty feeder pig is its expected slaughter grade at a market weight of 100kg after a normal feeding period. In these feeder pig standards, logical slaughter potential is determined by a composite appraisal of the development of the muscular system and the skeletal system. Both of these factors have an important effect on the development of lean and fat as the animal grows and fattens, and therefore, on the expected slaughter and carcass grade. Thriftiness in a feeder pig is its apparent ability to gain weight rapidly and efficiently. Size for age, health, and other general indications of thriftiness are considered in appraising the thriftiness of feeder pigs.

General criteria for selecting feeder pigs: They should be purchased from healthy herd. It should be vaccinated against major diseases. They should be free from any injury or wound. They should be extremely lean and muscular at purchase. The leanness should be maintained until they reach market age. Large-framed animals are desirable because they mature later and stay leaner at higher weights. Large-framed animals are taller, and the cannon bones in their front legs are longer than those of smaller-framed animals.

General criteria for selecting slaughter pigs: Lean meaty cuts, muscling, size or age and soundness are the important criteria for selecting pigs for slaughter. They must be mostly free from fat to produce lean pork. The loin should be narrower than its shoulder and ham regions. Heavily muscled market hogs produce more saleable pork than more lightly muscled hogs. Hogs should be evaluated for the expression, or definition, of muscle instead of pure thickness which may be due to fat.Market weight is usually between 110 and 120 kg, reached at an age of 5 to 6 months. Only healthy and sound animal should be selected.

13.2 Selection of Breeding Stock

Selecting productive and performance oriented breeding stock is the basic step for profitable swine production. Productive breeding stock is sound, fast growing, muscular, lean, and reproductively efficient. Breed choice depends on personal preference and availability in the area. Breeding animals should be evaluated for reproductive soundness, skeletal soundness, growth and potential production, frame size, and leanness and muscling. Superior animals excel in all these traits. Producers should never select animals on a single trait without considering the others.

13.2.1 Selection of Breeding Boars

Since producers usually select replacement gilts from their own herds, most of the genetic improvement will result from purchased boars. The selection and purchase of boars affects the economic wellbeing of a pork production enterprise. It is important to selected boars mainly from selected source which maintains records for the health, breed, performance and genetic improvement program. After going through these records, boars can be selected by considering soundness, sexual behavior and genetic merit. A boar must possess both the physical soundness to remain an active breeder, and the genetic potential to improve the performance of his progeny. In general, following factors should be considered for selecting breeding boars.

Health: New diseases are mainly brought on to farms by the introduction of pigs. It is important to select breeding stock from single supplier having improved health and genetic status of swine. Health history of the herd though record should also be done. It will reduce the risk of bringing in new diseases to the piggery. Disease status of a herd may be determined by clinical observation (eg. coughing, diarrhea, deaths, scratching); herd health records (growth and mortality); post-mortem results from pigs that have died on farm; medication records as many medications can mask disease symptoms; diagnostic tests undertaken on specimens submitted from pigs and conducted by laboratories with specialist pig expertise. Stock should be checked for swine dysentery, mange, mycoplasma pneumonia, pleuropneumonia atrophic rhinitis, worms, Glasser's disease, ileitis, colibacillosis, greasy pig disease, streptococcal meningitis, erysipelas and leptospirosis. Quarantine of new stock and acclimatization provides insurance against new diseases being introduced and allows new boars to be exposed and gain immunity to diseases on your unit.

Breed: It is important for tropics to buy such breed which are easily adaptive to given climate. Boars produced by comprehensive testing and improvement programs are recommended. Whether purebred or crossbred boars are used, select the breed appropriate to the crossbreeding system. The crossbreeding program will maintain high levels of heterosis and good pig survival. Crossbred boar use has become common in the more intensive production units. Research and producer experience indicate that crossbred boars are more aggressive breeders and produce higher farrowing rates than purebred boars. Fast growing lean boars that are sound and exhibit sexual aggressiveness are preferred.

Reproductive Efficiency: Although heritability of reproductive traits is low. However, selection of boars from higher litter size, number farrowed alive, birth weight, weaning weight are very important to profitable swine production. Select boars from large (8 or more weaned), healthy, problem-free litters. The reproductive tract is within the body and not visible, inspection of the external organs will give a good indication of reproductive soundness. Boars should be examined for testicle development. The testicles should be the larger in size with the epididymis prominent at the top of the scrotum. The testes should feel firm but not hard. If the testes are adequately developed and normal in appearance, the rest of the tract will probably be normal also. Behavioral patterns are important in selecting reproductive efficiency. Select breeding stock sired by considering sexually aggression and masculinity.

Soundness: Most hogs are raised indoors on concrete floors. They must be skeletally sound to survive, grow, and reproduce in confinement. Breeding stock must be structurally sound. They should have sloping shoulder, forearm, and pastern to serve as front shock absorbers.

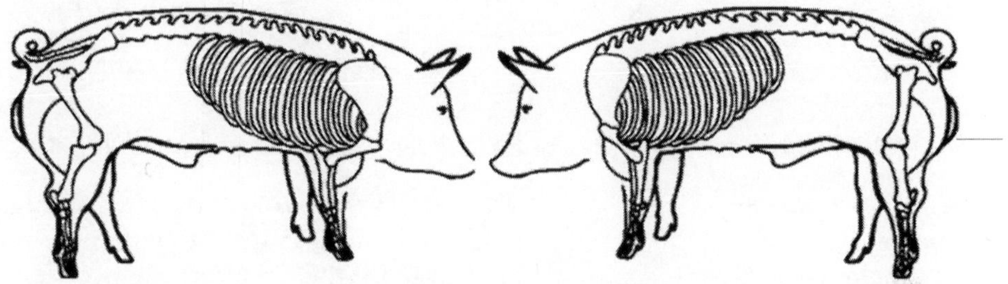

A: Desirable front and rear leg structure   B: Undesirable front and rear leg structure

Figure 13.1: Desirable front and rear leg structure (A) and undesirable front and rear leg structure (B)

Boar's legs and feet as they are subjected to considerable strain during mating. Unsoundness of feet and legs is the main problem encountered with young boars. Breeder's herd should be observed for signs of lameness, especially among market weight hogs. Any sign of weakness at early age could signal a serious problem at a later date. Make sure that his toes and pasterns are not long, weak or misshapen. When he walks, he should move freely, without any sign of stiffness or lameness. A level rump, high tail setting, and hock angulation are also important. Flexion (proper set to hock joint) for rear leg soundness should also be checked (Figure 13.1). A level top, moderate length of neck, and large, even-sized toes aid structural soundness. Boars should also be able to move with ease and must be sound to service sows.

Leanness: Since fat is neither economical to produce nor trim off the carcass, the selection of lean breeding stock is important. To produce lean and heavily muscled market hogs, breeding stock should be leaner and more muscular than average. Boars and gilts should be clean over their loin edge; their shoulder blades should be easily seen; and they should be free from excessive waste in the cushion of their hams. Back fat probes and ultrasonic instruments are useful to look at back fat and loin eye area, which are the best indicators ofleanness and muscularity. A large frame size is important in producing lean animals at high weights. Large-framed animals remain leaner at heavier weights than do small-framed animals. Figure 13.2 compares a trim, lean topped boar with a fat, wasty one.

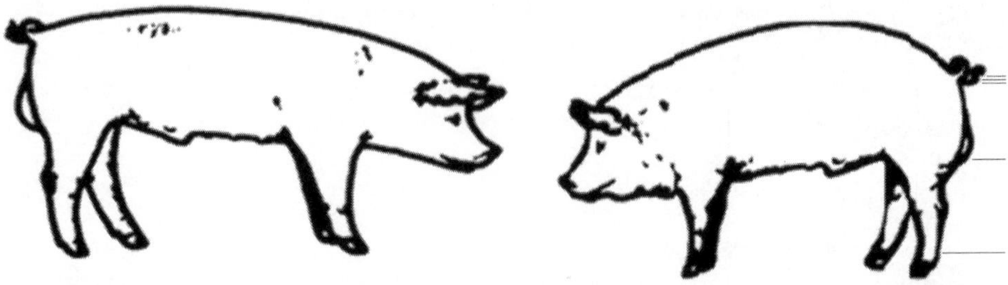

Fig 13.2: Trim and lean topped boar (left) and fat, round and wasty boar (right).

Growth Rate: Breeding boars should be selected for fast growth and high production. Growth records should be checked before purchase. If records are not available, select breeding stock that are large for their age, adequate in frame size, depth and capacity. A large body capacity allows animals to consume greater amounts of feed.

13.2.2 Selection of breeding gilt

The major goal of swine producers is to produce more live pigs per sow per year which can be achieved by increasing the size of individual litters born alive, increasing the number of times a sow farrows in a year. The size of litters is influenced by ovulation rate, conception rate, embryonic survival, lactation length, boar fertility and age of gilts at breeding. Since these factors are influenced greatly by genetics hence, proper selection of breeding gilt can give excellent financial return. Replacement gilt selection will vary greatly from farm to farm depending upon the crossbreeding system used and whether gilts are home raised or purchased. Regardless of source, fast growing lean gilts that are sound are preferred. Soundness of replacement gilts determined by functionality of skeleton, mammary and reproductive system. In general, following factors should be considered for selecting breeding gilts.

Health and breed: Consideration for health and breed during selection and purchase of gilt and boars are similar and discussed in selection of breeding boar section.

Soundness: Selected breeding stock must be structurally sound. Legs, feet and general conformation Gilts must possess sound legs and feet without any sign of weakness. Choose gilts which can move freely on their feet and legs and can function in the production facilities. Gilts should be wide through the hindquarters with depth and squareness in the body cavity. Sloping shoulder, forearm and pastern should serve as front shock absorbers. A level rump, high tail setting, and hock angulation are also important, and there must be flexion for rear leg soundness. A level top, moderate length of neck and large, even-sized toes are also important for structural soundness. The structural soundness and unsoundness of gilts are presented in figure 13.3. Unsound gilt shows straight in her shoulder, bucked over on her front legs, and steep and straight on her pasterns. She is also extremely high in her rump and post legged. These type of stock cannot stand the stress of breeding and farrowing and also lack long, productive life.

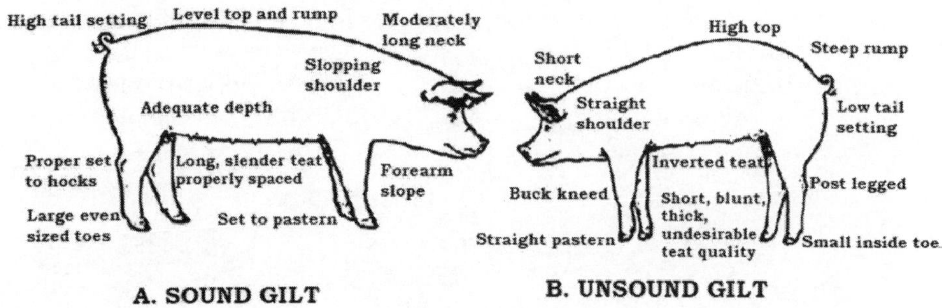

Figure 13.3: Features of sound and unsound gilt.

Growth Rate: As with boar selection, gilts should be selected on performance, namely growth rate and lean and fat composition. Fast growing breeding stock is a must. Since hogs that grow fast are usually more efficient (less feed per pound of gain), growth rate is very important. Growth records should be used to know about the growth rate. If records are not available, select breeding stock that are large for their age, moderate in frame size, and adequate in depth and capacity. Breeding gilts should be selected from large litters of pigs, because a sow that can raise a large litter has mothering ability, which is a desired trait. Various selection indices are available which take into consideration the prolificacy of sow lines and their ability to wean large numbers of heavy, healthy piglets. Replacement gilts are then drawn from these superior lines. They must also have an acceptable body capacity. A large body capacity allows animals to consume greater amounts of feed.

Mammary System: Underlines of gilts must be checked for both teat quality and number (figure 13.4). Choose replacement gilts with an adequate number of apparently functional teats to wean large litters. Gilts should possess at least seven evenly spaced teats on either side. They should start well forward and be in a straight line. Desirable nipples are long, narrow, and well defined. Problems such as poor spacing, blind, scarred (teat necrosis) and inverted teats should be avoided.

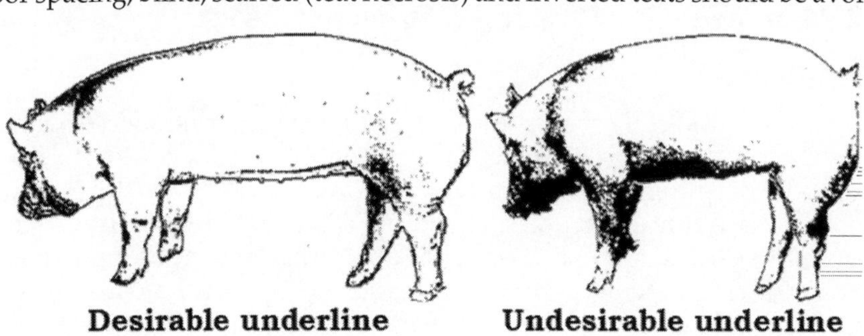

Figure 13.4: Desirable and undesirable underlines in gilts.

Reproductive System: Choose gilts with normal appearing external genetalia. Most of the reproductive organs are internal and not visible. Normal development of external genetalia is the best indicator of a sound reproductive system. Increased prominence of the vulva and mammary system as the gilt nears puberty is a good indication of development of a normal reproductive system. With visual selection the only reliable feature that can be accounted for is the shape, size and placement of the vulva. It should be large, without sign of infantilism, and free of the 'fish hook' appearance found in hermaphrodites (figure 13.5).

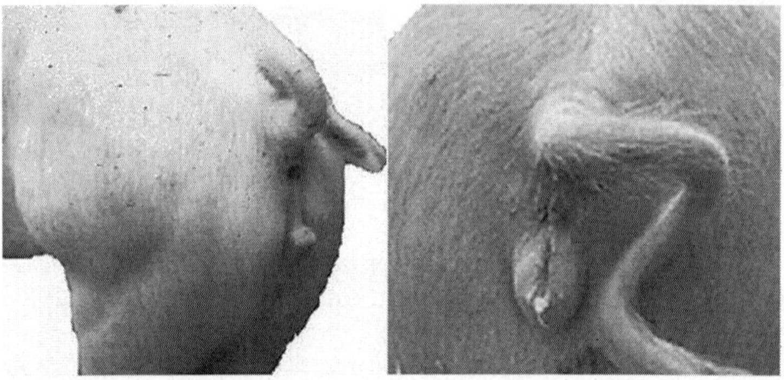

A. Fish hook appearance of vulva in hermaphrodites **B. Normal vulva of gilt**

Figure 13.5: Fish hook appearance of vulva in hermaphrodites and normal vulva of gilt.

Reproductive Efficiency: Although heritability of reproductive traits is low. However, selection of gilts from higher litter size, number farrowed alive, birth weight, weaning weight are very important to profitable swine production. Select gilts from large (8 or more weaned), healthy, problem-free litters. Temperament of gilts should be quiet but alert and active. If there is any tendency to be flighty or overly aggressive, they should be disregarded as future breeders. While management plays an important part in the development of certain behaviors, many problems at farrowing time could be averted by careful selection of gilt replacements.

13.3 Management of Selected Breeding Stock

Quarantine

Selected stocks are the main source of new diseases to be introduced in to farms. Isolation and quarantine are the major steps to control introduction to new diseases. The purpose of quarantine is to protect the main herd against the introduction of new infectious agents that cause economically damaging disease. Health status of the incoming stock should be thoroughly done. They should be dewormed and treated for lice and mange. Then they should be vaccinated against erysipelas, leptospirosis and parvovirus. The ideal quarantine housing would be far away from old stock. The new stock of pigs should be cleaned, disinfected prior to occupation by newly purchased stock. Any feed, equipment and vehicles present on the main farm would not enter or leave the quarantine area without thorough cleaning and disinfection. Use separate boots and protective clothing when working with animals in quarantine. Provide a draft-free sleeping area with ample supply of fresh water. Watch for signs of illness throughout the isolation period. If in doubt about the swine dysentery or spiröchetal status of the supplier herd then they should be medicated for two week period before allowing them into the herd.

13.4 Routine Vaccination Programs for Gilts/Sows and Boars

Vaccination is the best prophylaxis measure against disease. A number of vaccines are available for routine use in pig herds. The vaccination program starts immediately after selection but full protection comes only two weeks after the booster dose. Combination vaccines are now available. Routine vaccination against erysipelas, leptospirosis, parvovirus and E coli should be considered when introducing young gilts to the herd. When naïve animals are introduced into a herd with endemic disease, other vaccines are recommended. These include Mycoplasma, Glasser's disease, proliferative enteritis and pleuropneumonia vaccines. Leptospirosis, parvovirus and erysipelas boosters must be given before mating to ensure adequate protection for the developing fetuses. With E coli vaccinations, the objective is to produce maximum antibody levels in the gilt's colostrum at her first farrowing. The booster for E coli must be given 3 weeks before farrowing. The primary injection can be given at selection, or as late as 4 weeks before the booster shot.Booster vaccinations should be given for erysipelas and leptospirosis about 3 weeks before farrowing (table 13.1). This will boost antibody levels in the sow's colostrum, giving additional protection to the litter, as well as providing protection to the sow for her next pregnancy.

Table 13.1: Vaccination schedule for new unmated gilts

	Leptospirosis	*Erysipelas*	*Optional for Actinobacillus pleuropneumoniae& Glasser's disease*	*E coli*	*Parvovirus*
At selection	+	+		+	+
2-4 weeks later	+	+	+		+
2-3 weeks before farrowing (gilts)	+	+	+	+	
2-3 weeks before farrowing (sows)	+	+		+	+

❑❑❑

Chapter 14

Systems of Breeding

—Dr. Niraj Kumar

There are various methods of breeding for swine herd. The choice of system of breeding is determined by many factors like size of herd, quality of herd, infrastructure, management and goal of the farm. There is no one best system of breeding or secret of success for any and all conditions. For example, to produce breeding or commercial stock systems of breeding are quite different. Following are some of the common breeding systems used commonly in swine farm. Broadly, the system of breeding is of two types i.e. inbreeding and out breeding.

14.1 Inbreeding

This means the mating of related individuals. Relationship becomes a vague term and must be specified. So in order to be more specific we should say that inbreeding involves the mating of related individuals within 4-6 generations. It has also been defined as the mating of more closely related individuals than the average if the population. Inbreeding can again be divided into close breeding and line breeding.

(a) Close breeding

Mating between individuals of the same breed but which are more closely related than the average of the breed. This means the mating of full sister to full brother or sire to his daughter or dam to her son. These types of mating should be used only when both parents are outstanding individuals. The major objective of pure-breeding is to identify and propagate superior genes for use in commercial production primarily in crossbreeding programs as well as to propagate and identify superior females for maintaining valuable genetic material. Crossbreeding will not be worthwhile unless superior pure bred individuals are used. The effect of inbreeding is the concentration of common genes in the offspring. This high frequency of homozygous gene pairs applies to both desirable and undesirable traits. Many undesirable traits e.g. hernia and cryptorchidism involve recessive genes thus inbreeding perpetuates their expression phenotypically.

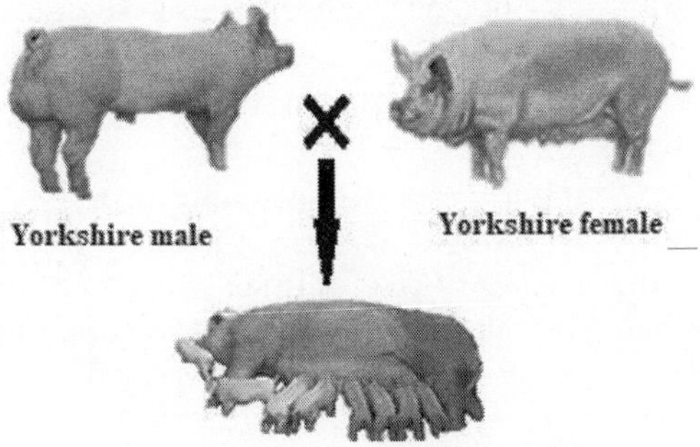

Figure 14.1: Mating between closely related Yorkshire male and female (close breeding)

The advantage of close breeding is that, undesirable recessive genes may be discovered and eliminated by further testing in this line. The progeny are more uniform than outbred progeny. Mating between closely related Yorkshire male and female are shown in Figure 14.1.

(b) Line breeding

The mating of animals of wider degrees of relationship than those selected for close breeding. It promotes uniformity in character. Homozygosity is not reached so quickly as in close breeding. Neither desirable nor harmful characters are developed so quickly as in close breeding. It is a showed method for the fixation of hereditary outstanding boar or saw and the progeny is mentioned as being line bred to certain ancestors. It is usually directed towards keeping the offspring related to some highly prized ancestor. Linebreeding is practiced to conserve desirable traits of an outstanding boar or sow line.

In breeding causes decrease in litter size and increases mortality. Inbred sows are inferior in milking and mothering ability. It delays sexual maturity in gilts and boars. Inbred boars have less sexual libido. Inbred gilts have fewer eggs during oestrus and farrow smaller litters than those out bred. Inbreeding is suggested for only highly qualified operators who are making an effort to stabilize important traits in a given set of animals. Intensive selection is needed to reduce the risk of producing undesirable traits in breeding stock when inbreeding is practiced.

14.2 Out-breeding

Out-breeding is the breeding of unrelated animals. It consists of various kinds of mating like out-crossing and cross-breeding. Cross breeding can be done in various ways like criss- crossing, triple crossing, two or three breed rotational crossing depending on the need of the producer.

(a) Outcrossing

It consists of the practice of mating of unrelated pure bred animals within the same breed. The animals mated have no common ancestors on either side of their side of their pedigree up to 4-6 generations and the offspring of such a mating is known as the out-crossing. This is the general system that is practiced by most purebred breeders and is classified as a safe system in the purebred business. This method is highly effective for characters that are largely under the control of genes with additive effects. It is an effective system for genetic improvement if carefully combined with selection.

(b) Cross breeding

Crossbreeding is the mating of two animals which are members of different breeds. This system is being practiced by the majority of commercial swine producers because of the resulting hybrid vigor that makes possible improved production efficiency. Mating two individuals from different breeds thus introducing into the progeny a gene combination that is different from that existing in either parent or in the breed of either parent. Crossbreeding can be a very useful tool for the pork producer to increase the efficiency and profit of an operation. Full benefits from crossbreeding can be gained only by careful combination of available breeds and selection of outstanding breeding animal replacements from within those breeds. Crossbreeding programs must be systematic and well-planned to take full advantage of heterosis and breed differences. Crossbreeding enables the producer to take advantage of heterosis and to combine desirable characteristics of different breeds. Heterosis is the difference between crossbred animals and the average of their purebred counterparts. Desirable characteristics of different breeds can be utilized if some breeds can be identified as good maternal breeds and others as good paternal breeds. A system where males from paternal breeds (superior growth and carcass) are mated to females from maternal breeds (superior reproduction and mothering ability) can take advantage of the strengths of both breeds while minimizing some of the weaknesses. Two basic systems exist, each of which has several variations. They can also be used in combination. These are the rotational cross system and the terminal cross system. Rotational cross systems combine two or more breeds, where the breed of boar used is different from the previous generation and replacement crossbred females are retained from each cross. The major difference is that rotational cross replacement females are produced within the system while terminal cross female replacements are usually purchased or produced by maintaining purebred herds that emphasize reproductive performance.

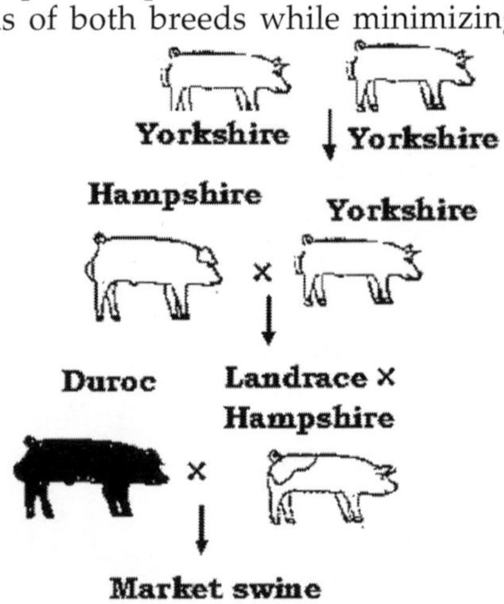

Figure 14.2: Terminal cross of Duroc boars and Hampshire x Yorkshire cross females

(i) Terminal Cross Systems

This systems may involve two, three, or four breeds. A two-breed cross will utilize purebred boars on one breed mated to purebred sows of another breed. For example, Hampshire boars and Yorkshire females could be used to produce every pig crop. The attempt here is to capitalize on the muscling traits of the Hampshire, mothering ability of the Yorkshire. A three-breed terminal cross will utilize purebred boars of one breed mated to crossbred sows of two other breeds. For example Duroc boars and Hampshire x Yorkshire cross females could be used to produce each pig crop (figure 14.2). The attempt here is to capitalize on the muscling traits of the Hampshire, mothering ability of the York and the growth ability of the Duroc or any such combination of breeds which suits the producer's need.

Crossbred sows are utilized so that this system maximizes heterosis and is expected to be one of the most productive systems. A four-breed terminal cross has all of the same advantages on the maternal side as the three-breed cross. In addition, there are some advantages in conception rate associated with use in crossbred boars. In general, terminal crosses capitalize on the strengths of each breed and realize maximum gains from heterosis. A big disadvantage of terminal crosses can be the difficulty of obtaining replacement females.

(ii) Rotation Cross Systems

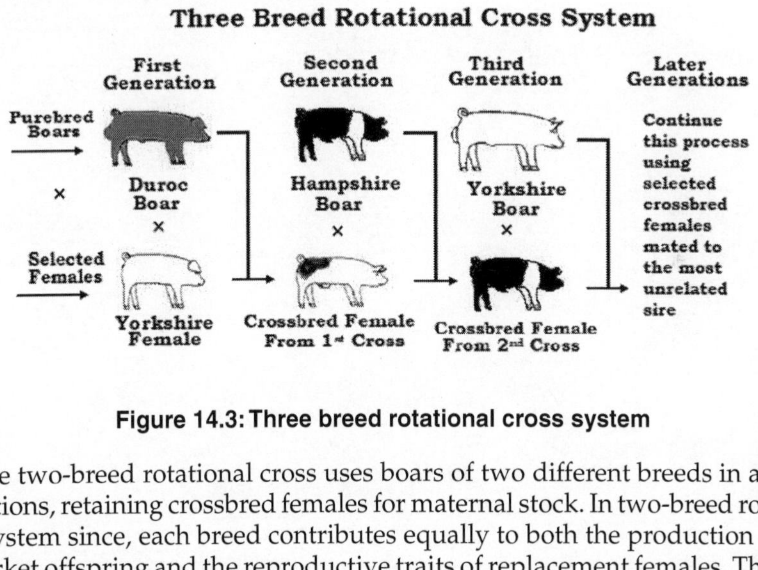

Figure 14.3: Three breed rotational cross system

The two-breed rotational cross uses boars of two different breeds in alternate generations, retaining crossbred females for maternal stock. In two-breed rotational cross system since, each breed contributes equally to both the production traits of the market offspring and the reproductive traits of replacement females. Therefore, reproductively sound breeds with adequate growth and carcass characteristics should be used. More heterosis can be realized with the addition of a third breed to the rotation. Three breed rotations (figure 14.3) are recommended over two-breed rotations, since a higher percentage of the total advantage obtained from crossbreeding is realized. The number of breeding groups that need to be maintained also increases with the number of breeds included in the rotation since females of different parities will be at different stages of the rotation and will require different breeds of boars or mates. The rotation cross system is more popular and thought by many to be a more practical program than the terminal cross system. This is because the only outside breeding stock that needs to be purchased, once the program is established, are boars. Thus a producer does not have the difficulty of obtaining replacement females at a reasonable cost. Combinations of desirable traits of breeds cannot be fully utilized in a rotational system. Ideally, market hogs should be out of sows with good mothering ability and sired by boars that excel in growth and carcass characteristics. This is difficult to achieve in the framework of a rotational crossing system.

Chapter 15

Piglet Management - Birth to Weaning

— Dr. Niraj Kumar & Mr. Tsegay Tkue

Proper care and management during farrowing has a significant role to improve survival and well-being of the newborn pigs. It will also enhance the number of live born piglets that are weaned and improve perform in later stages of production. Prior to farrowing, the saws should be treated for external and internal parasite to keep the newborn pigs free of lice, ticks, and worms. Vaccination should also be done in order to pass the immunity to the piglets. Most common vaccination programs include treatment for scours and respiratory diseases. Usually, saw are transferred to clean and disinfected farrowing pen three to five to five days prior to expected date of farrowing.

15.1 Behaviour of Saw During Farrowing

The saw will appear nervous one day prior to farrowing. They may exhibit sign of nest building by thumping front feet to the ground. The small amount of straw may be provided to satisfy the nest building desire. Ten to twelve hours before, milk will appear in the udder in saw. Gilts may not show signs of milk. Two to six hours before the onset of birth of first piglet, labor will begin and the sow's respiration rate will increase. Generally farrowing will last within one to four hours after the birth of first piglet. The duration of farrowing depends on the litter size and the parity. Expulsion of placental membrane is the signal for farrowing to be over.

15.2 Mortality in piglets

Generally 10-15% mortality is common in piglet from birth to weaning. Birth weights are a critical factor in piglet survival and they are the one at most risk. Around half of these losses occur mostly from piglets having least body weight in the litter. First three days after the birth are more critical and around two-third deaths occur during this period. The weak piglets may die due to hunger when they fail to suckle because of low viability or low birth weight. The length of farrowing may affect the number of piglets born dead or with a reduced ability to survive. This is often caused by damage to the umbilical cord during birth and the resulting partial or complete asphyxiation. Farrowing may slow down during hot weather or when sows are too fat or constipated.

Lightweight piglets are weakened by the rigors of the birth process, and may have a congenital defect(s) like splay leg. These piglets are not able to get on their feet and to the udder. They cannot compete with stronger, normal litter mates for access to teats during the first hours after birth. This reduces their intake of colostrum. Normal piglets will be born quickly, get on their feet and start suckling immediately. They move from teat to teat, taking a disproportionately large share of the most concentrated, immunoglobulin-rich colostrum. It is essential that the piglets get the passive immunity provided in the colostrum because very little transfer of antibodies across the placenta prior to birth. Piglets contain fat energy in their body for about one day of life, and they cannot regulate internal body temperature well until they are a few days old. Chilling often experience a lower core body temperature which makes them susceptible to death. Often these piglets are seen shivering and huddled with litter mates, because their thermal requirements have not been met.

15.3 Assistance during farrowing

Adequate observation and assistance could save more pigs born alive. This could add another 2-3 pigs per sow a year, resulting in a large increase in net return per sow. Assistance is required during prolonged labor and difficult birth due to oversized and malpositioned piglets that obstruct the birth canal. Gentle pulling may be beneficial to facilitate farrowing and to save lives of the piglets. Some piglets may be born with their snouts covered by fetal membrane and showing no movement and seems to be dead. After removing fetal membrane from mouth and nostrils to clear respiratory tract and giving massage or mouth to mouth resuscitation with funnel or swinging may revive the piglets. Weak piglets should be helped to find the sow's teats for suckling.

15.4 Prevent Chilling

Chilling is one of the most important cause of piglet mortality. The newborn piglets are extremely susceptible to cold, damp conditions. Chilling makes piglet weak and sluggish, leaving it vulnerable to other dangers such as crushing and starvation and predisposes them to diarrhea (scouring) and respiratory infections. The first five days are critical to piglet survival because they cannot regulate their body temperature. Also, they have little fat and hair, a thin skin and a small mass in relation to its body surface area. Piglets are born with a limited supply of readily available energy and must suckle shortly after birth to maintain their blood sugar levels to prevent them from death. Cold conditions force piglets to use up these reserves very quickly, and, when weakened, the piglet has less chance of survival. To prevent chilling, quickly dry newborn piglets and clear their lungs of mucus. Keep the piglets dry when bathing the sow or cleaning the pen.

The farrowing area requires two different microclimates. Sow needs relatively cool area with temperature range 60-65 F while the newborn piglets requires 85-95 F the first few days, then decreased to the 70-80 F range until weaning. The temperature of farrowing room should be maintained at approximately 65-70 F and heating zone should be provided to the litter. The heated area for the piglets should be away from the sow. High temperature in the farrowing area decreases the feed intake and milk production on saw. The heat source will attract the piglets and reduce the incidence of crushing. Closely monitor the sow and litter's responses to the zone heating to ensure their thermal needs are met. Observe the behavior of the piglets. If they are too cold, they will pile up under the heat source; if they are too warm, they will stay away from the heat source. Very small, weak and piglets with splay legs should be kept in a crib which is a dry box with a thermostatically controlled heater lamp. Here, they kept away from saw to receive required temperature they need and are protected from being crushed by the sow. They can be bottle fed or stomach tubed, and, when recovered, placed back on the sow.

15.5 Colostrum feeding

Colostrum is the first flow of milk produced by the sow after giving birth. It is rich in fat and protein and it contains antibodies that help protect the baby pigs against common infections and diseases until they can produce their own antibodies at 3-4 weeks of age. The concentration of immunoglobulins in the very first colostrum is very high which declines over time. Immunoglobulins from colostrum are absorbed in higher amount into bloodstream immediately after birth. The absorption declines soon hence, they must consume as much colostrum as possible within the first few hours. Piglets that do not consume colostrum milk have a low survival rate and are susceptible to diseases. To ensure weak or deprived piglets receive adequate quantities of colostrum they can be bottle fed with colostrum collected from the sow while she is farrowing. If all the colostrum is not required that day, it can be frozen then reheated to body temperature when needed. Cow colostrum also can be used and may more easily obtained. Collected colostrum can be bottle fed to piglets or given via a stomach tube or a syringe. Small piglets will need 20–30 ml every 2 hours or so until they are mobile. Split suckling is useful when only one sow is available in a large litter. Put the large piglets in a warm box (crib) for one hour three times a day to give the smaller ones a chance to nurse without competition, or split the litter into two groups and alternate their suckling time. Split suckling improves the survival and growth rates of smaller piglets. If the sow dies at parturition or suffers from "no-milk syndrome," foster piglets to other newly-farrowed sows.

15.6 Fostering

Cross-fostering is the distribution of piglets among different sows. It is the most effective way to reduce within-litter piglet weight variation. Piglets need to be fostered to other sows when a sow had a large litter of healthy pigs and not enough functional teats, orphaned piglets or litters from sows afflicted with agalactia (no milk production after farrowing) or a saw with large litter with uneven sized piglets. When sows and gilts farrow in batches, it is possible to equalize litters and adjust litter size to the number of functioning teats or to the nursing ability of the sows. The survival of small or weak piglets is improved if they are nursed as a group separately from large piglets. Ensure piglets that will be cross fostered consume colostrum from their dam. Allow piglets to remain with their dam for at least four to six hours following birth before they are cross fostered. Otherwise, it is likely the fostered piglets will not consume an adequate amount of colostrum, especially if they are fostered to a sow which farrowed one to two days previously. There is a risk that the sow will not accept any of the piglets to be transferred. To avoid rejection, the piglets to be transferred can be almost immediately rubbed in the gleanings or urine of the sow to which they are to be transferred. Where this is not possible, remove the piglets to be transferred and the litter they are to be matched with, and place them together in a box under a heat lamp before placing them with the sow. Some success can be obtained by masking the odor of the pigs by some strong-smelling substance.

15.7 Orphan pigs

When a sow or gilt dies or dries-off and there is no chance of fostering piglets, an attempt can be made to raise them artificially. Raising such pigs is time-consuming. Feeding colostrum either from cow or other source is important. Commercial milk replacer products should be used to raise orphan pigs. When hand fed, they can be fed 40–50 ml for four to six times per day and then increased up to 80–100 ml per feed. Overfeeding piglets will increase susceptibility to scouring. If piglets orphaned at 1 week old or later, they can be placed on liquid diets for the first few days and then switched to dry meals (milk based).

15.8 Piglet husbandry practices

15.8.1 Cutting the umbilical cord

During pregnancy, the unborn pig receives nutrients and voids body waste through the umbilical cord. During farrowing, as the piglet comes out and the umbilical cord breaks, but the remaining navel cord can be an entry for pathogens into the piglet's body. Cut the cord 1 inch from the base and dip the stump in iodine. To avoid piglet infections, do not leave the umbilical cord uncut or without disinfectant. If the cord does not break naturally, wait 5-10 minutes after the piglet comes out and pull the cord gently until it breaks. If excess bleeding occurs from the umbilical cord, tie it off immediately with string or clamp the stump with forceps for 1-2 minutes. Then apply iodine antiseptic by swabbing, spraying, or dipping.

15.8.2 Removal of needle teeth

Piglets are born with eight sharp and small teeth (two on each side, top and bottom) that could injure the sow's teats and the faces of other piglets during suckling. Clipping one-half of teeth off at birth with sharp cutter pliers is required. Care should be taken for not to damage the tongue or gums. The teeth can be cut off using a strong pair of disinfected sharp cutters without nicks in the blades. It is not recommended to remove entire tooth and avoid crushing or breaking of teeth. Teeth should be cut off flat and not at an angle. Piglets will not cause skin injuries when they fight if the teeth are cut off flat. Do not remove the entire tooth and avoid crushing or breaking it. Otherwise, an infection is possible or the piglet may not nurse well.

15.8.3 Tail docking

As pigs come in close contact with each other they may attempt to bite or chew the tail of their pen mates. The causes of tail biting are behavioral or stress factors. Overcrowding, poor environment, severe restriction of feed, poorly balanced rations and a high incidence of external parasites are some common stress factors. When tail biting is a problem, all aspects should be investigated. The loss of the pig's tail is of no commercial significance, but it can lead to infection through biting and complications may arise. It can seriously affect growth rates and result in the death of pigs or condemnations of affected pigs at the abattoir. Tail docking should be done within the first two days after birth because the piglets are small, easier to hold and less stressful at this stage. Also, the littermates are less likely to bite at the wound on the docked tail at this age. The tail should be cut one inch from the base with a pair of sterilized scissors or side cutters. Cutting the tail too short could interfere with muscle activity around the anus later in the piglet's life and could be an aggravating factor in rectal prolapse or rear leg paralysis. If too much tail is left, tail biting might still occur. Occasionally, a tail will bleed excessively. If this occurs, tie it off using the string. Apply an antiseptic to the wound. The tail should be completely healed within 7-10 days. Piglets chosen for breeding stock should not have their tails cut. Breeding animals use their tails to drive flies away from the vulva when secretions are present during estrus and farrowing. Intact tails in boars and sows also give them a better appearance.

15.8.4 Identification in pigs

Pigs require permanent identification for management records. Each piglet must have a unique ear notch or tattoo in seed stock herds because it is a requirement for pedigree and performance records. Performance of finishers can be easily traced to sows and boars that have been properly identified. Several methods may be used such as ear notching, ear tattooing, electronic transponders, or ear tags. Pigs can be permanently identified by notching or tattooing their ears.

Ear Tags: Plastic tags are commonly used for replacement and breeding animals. They are easy to read even at a distance. There are varying shapes and types of ear tags. Some tags are pre-numbered, others are supplied blank and can be numbered with a special pen. These tags are attached to the piglet's ear by using special applicator pliers. Numbered ear tags are not usually suitable for pigs penned together as the tags can be lost during playing or fighting with pen mates.

Ear tattooing: Ear tattooing is done in piglets when they are 2-3 weeks old. The equipment required is a set of tattoo pliers, three or four sets of 9 mm needle blocks numbered from 0 to 9 and a suitable tattooing ink or paste. The thinner part of the lower ear (inside or outside) is most suitable for tattooing and are cleaned properly. Proper digits are placed in the pliers and apply pressure to the piglet's ear until the digit marks are visible. The needles should completely pierce the pig's ear, avoiding veins where possible. Smear ink on the digit marks to produce a tattoo. Ear tattoos are mainly used in landrace and large white herds and in some commercial piggeries. This method is not very efficient as tattoos can be hard to read even when correctly done. Ear tattoo equipment (pliers and numerals) is more expensive than ear notching pliers and most commercial pig farmers find ear notching a suitable method of identification.

Ear notching: Ear notching should be performed within the first week of age. When done at this age, ear notching may be the least traumatic means of identification. Ear-notched pigs can be easily identified from a short distance and the notching remains visible for the life of the pig.

The most common ear notching system is that the litter number is notched in the piglet's right ear and the individual piglet number in the piglet's left ear (figure 15.1). Several modifications of the system exist. Use a V-ear notcher designed for piglets to ear notch. Notching should be done with care and considerations. Notches that are too shallow may fill in, heal over, and be difficult to read. Leave at least one-fourth inch between notches. Notches at the base of pigs' ears need to be cut deeper otherwise they may grow over in time. Do not make notches too close to the tip of the ear, as these can be torn off.

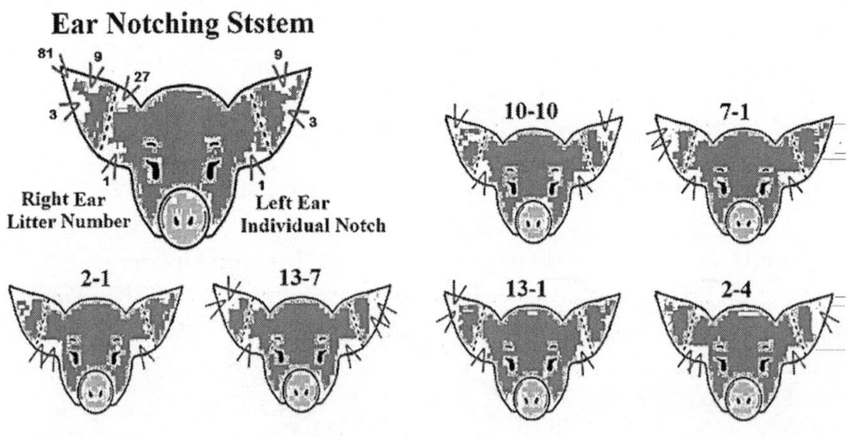

Figure 15.1: Identification of pig by ear notching. Right ear notch represent litter number while left ear notch represent individual pig number.

15.8.5 Castration

The surgical removal of the two testicles. It is a routine management practice for male pigletsnot selected for breeding purposes and raised for slaughter. The operation is less of a shock and the wound heals faster when the pigs are young. It should be done at early age preferably within one week after birth. Castration is needed to facilitate safe handling, good management, and to ensure carcass quality. Intact males become extremely aggressive as they approach puberty. Increased aggressiveness results in disruption and fighting within the herd or group and increases danger to the animal handler. In addition, meat from boars has an objectionable odor caused by an increase of male sex hormone levels in the intact male which becomes more pronounced when the meat is heated during cooking. It can be done by scalpel method or side cutter method.

Scalpel method: Piglets are restrained properly and the scrotal area disinfected with iodine. Then piglets are examined carefully before castrating to identify those with a scrotal hernia. Castrate should be avoided unless the person trained to repair hernias. Both testicles are then pushed up and an incision is given through the skin toward the tail through scrotal midline.

They are exposed by cutting through the membrane that separates them. Testicles are then popped up through the incision and pulled out slightly. After pulling out the testicles, cut the chords. Wound disinfectant is applied over the incisions after taking out the testicles (figure 15.2: a, b, c, d, e and f). In case of excessive bleeding the cord should be clamped or tied if bleeding persists.

Side-cutter method: This method is advantageous than scalpel method as there is less bleeding as blood vessels are pinched rather than sliced. Pigs are retrained properly. Testis is pushed up to make it more pronounced. The fold of skin is formed where the incision is made. Position side-cutters approximately two-third of the way into the fold and make a clean cut directly through the scrotal tissue right of the middle. Make another cut to the left of the midline. Then testicles are popped up, grasped and cords are pulled up slowly. With the help of index finger, it is ensured that the cord will break off at the point of index finger. There is no cutting of the cords in this method. Iodine is sprayed on the incision to prevent infection. Castrated pigs into clean pens free from dust, dirt or mud as they often lead to the formation of abscesses in the wounds.

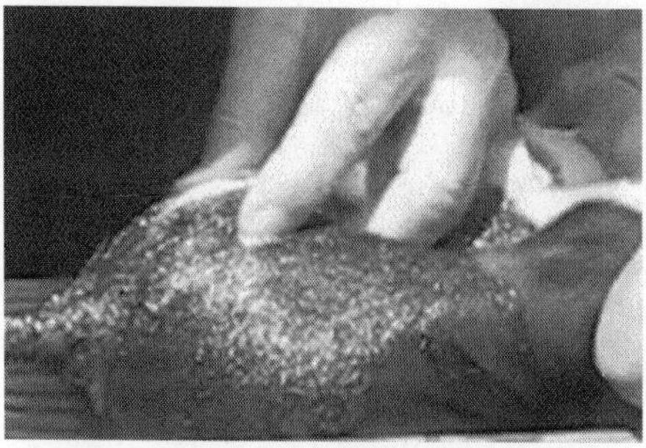

Figure 15.2 (a): Incision across the scrotal midline.

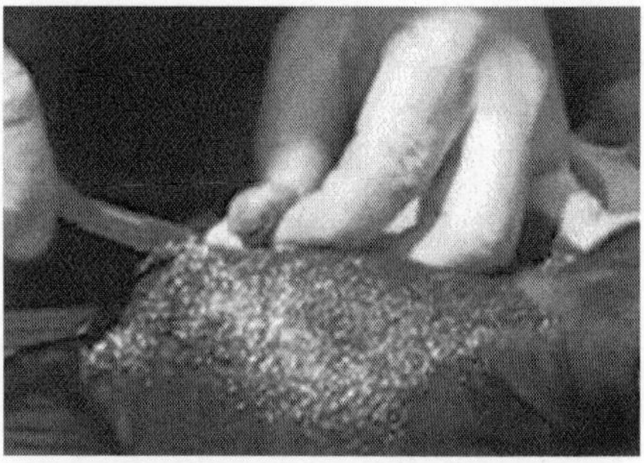

Figure 15.2 (b): Popping out the testicles.

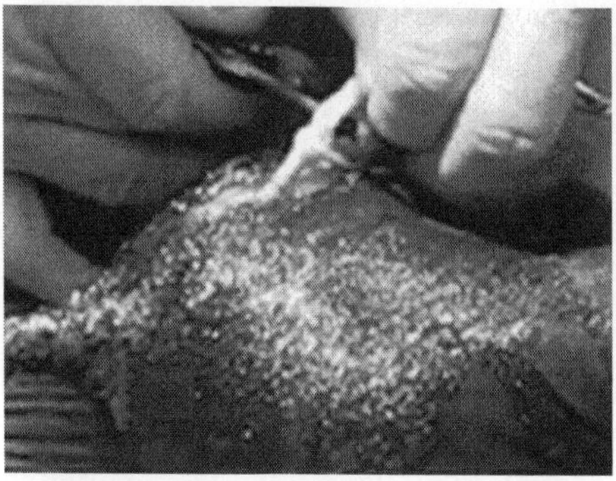

Figure 15.2 (c): Cutting of spermatic testicles.

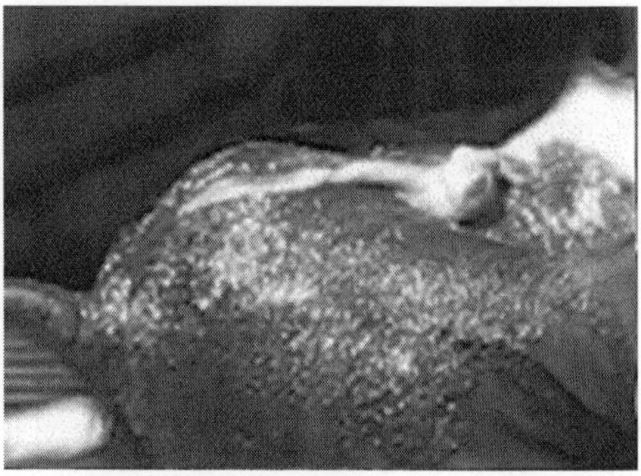

Figure 15.2 (d): Other testis outside the sac.

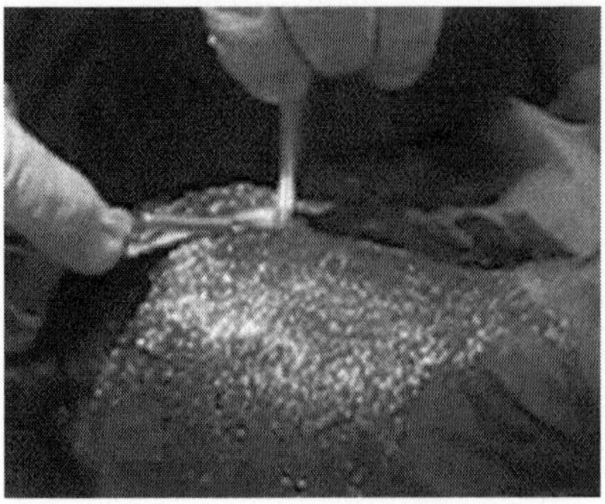

Figure 15.2 (e): Cutting of spermatic testicles.

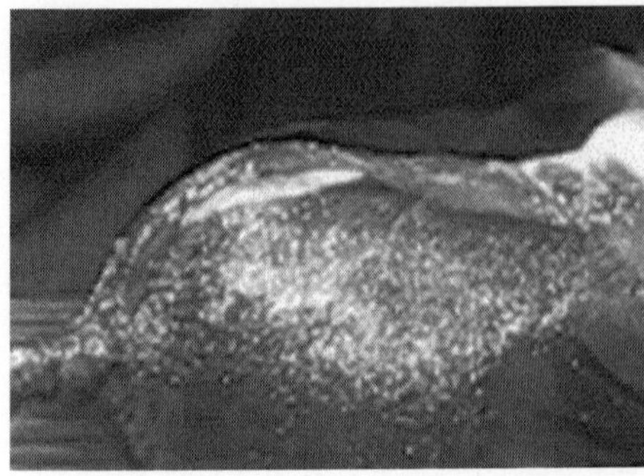

Figure 15.2 (f): Application of iodine

15.8.6 Piglet anemia

Anemia develops rapidly in nursing piglets because of low iron reserves in the newborn piglet, the low iron in sow's colostrum and milk and the lack of contact with iron in the soil. Piglets grows very quickly and its blood increases rapidly in volume. Consequently, it must have an adequate supply of iron. When a piglet is born, it has iron reserve in the body which last within 3–7 days and anemia may result in 7-10 days.

Affected Piglets will show heavy, jerky breathing and general weakness. The mucous membranes of the eyes and mouth become white in color and the skin loses its bright pink color. As the condition progresses, they pass a white, pasty scour. Unless iron is obtained from another source, the pigs will die. In the wild, pigs get iron by eating soil or manure. However, in modern farrowing areas the producer must provide iron by different sources.

Iron may be given to the piglets individually in a powdered reduced form, but an injectable iron dextrin compound is better. This should be injected intramuscularly at 3 days of age. Use a dosage of 150-200 mg. Injected form of iron should be given into the neck muscle just off the midline. Iron should not be injected into the ham. The injection should be given in the neck because of possible sciatic nerve damage, scarring, and also, because of residual iron stain in the carcass of market hogs if it is given in the ham. A second dose at 2-3 weeks of age may be needed if the piglets are eating very little creep feed. Various oral mixtures of iron can be used and are placed on the back of the tongue. These are best given within 36 hours of birth to be effective. Iron can also be provided in piglets' drinking water, with a dispenser placed in the creep area. Sow teat can be painted with iron sulfate paste every 2–3 days.

15.8.7 Management of Splay legged piglets

Splay legged piglets get difficulty to stand on their leg. When they attempt to stand, their hind legs (mainly) or forelegs extend sideways. The important predisposing factors for splay leg are either congenital, shorter gestation period or slippery floor of farrowing pen. If not assisted, these piglets are not able to suckle colostrum and they may die. Taping the legs together in correct position with duct tapes until the piglet recovers from the condition is effective. The tape is wrapped around the left back leg to up around the right ham over the back then down over the left ham and then around the right back leg prevents the leg from sliding outward. This tape is left for around one week or may be removed when piglets are able to stand or walk without assistance. Precaution should be taken not to wrap the tape too tightly as to restrict blood circulation.

15.8.8 Crushing of piglets

Crushing of piglets by the sow is one of the major reason of injuries and deaths during first week after birth. Farrowing crates are the best way to prevent crushing. Sow are placed in farrowing crate 2-4 days earlier to accustom to new environment. These crates will not allow the sow to move and to lie down on her belly before turning on her side and the chances of crushing the piglets are greatly reduced. Commercial metallic farrowing crates are available but it can be made by locally available material like wood, bamboo or iron rod as per the size of the saw.

15.8.9 Creep Feeding

Creep feeding (Pre starter ration) is recommended from two weeks of age until weaning. In saw, peak milk yield is achieved between 2-3 weeks and then it declines. As piglets are growing rapidly during early age and then tend to outstrip the nutrients provided by the sow's milk, and thus need supplementing. Then provision of special feed mixture inside a creep area is necessary. It should be readily available to the piglets but beyond the reach of the sow.

It is very difficult for the piglets to digest solid fibrous feed during first two weeks of age as their digestive system is not well developed. But at the age of 2-3 weeks, they are able to digest starch, sugars and non-milk protein in dry form. It also helps in reducing weaning stress, minimizing the effect of variation in milk consumption and improving the weaning weight of piglets. Small amounts of fresh feed should be provided in a shallow pan and increase the amount when the piglets start eating it. In farm formulation or commercial pre-starter rations containing 18-21% crude protein may be used as a creep feed. Potable water (nipple waterers) should be provided at all times.

❑❑❑

Chapter 16

Farrowing Management in Sows

—Dr. Awot Teklu

16.1 Farrowing management

The average gestation period of sows ranges 112-115 days. However, slightly lower or higher gestation values might occur based on the genetic and management differences among animals. Dilation of the cervix and movement of the fetus towards the opening of the cervix are of the typical indicator signs of parturition in sows. The entire process of farrowing is conventionally classified into three basic stages as discussed here after.

The preparatory/initiation stage

This stage is about 10-12 hours before the farrowing process took place. Some of the sighs seen at this time include restlessness, uneasy, hyperpnoea, nesting behaviors, and distention of the mammary glands. As parturition approaches more, the fetus will move to the opening of the cervix and this will be followed by uterine muscle contraction, breakage of the placental membrane, and expulsion of the amniotic fluid through the vulva, often known as the meconium. In general, the expulsion of the meconium (sometimes blood-stained) is an indication that delivery will follow soon within two hours period.

For a proper delivery and good performance of newborns, it is often recommended to use hormones to control farrowing in sows. The use of prostaglandins is often reported to cause dilation of the cervix by enhancing the release of relaxin. Furthermore, prostaglandin is also believed to stimulate the release of oxytocin into the circulation causing uterine muscle contraction and facilitating the expulsion of the newborns. Therefore, they are properly and appropriately used, prostaglandin and/or oxytocin injections can yield in normal and timely delivery of the pigs. Dosage wise, prostaglandin F2 should be prescribed at 10 mg at the 110th day of pregnancy or afterwards which will be effective at about 30 hours post injection. Similarly, oxytocin given at about 2 ml intramuscularly is reported to cause normal delivery too.

The delivery stage

The continuous muscular contractions end up with the expulsion of the protruding fetus out through the vulva. Normal delivery is associated with the exit of the hind legs or the nose of the newborn first. Piglets that come out first do often have higher chance of suckling colostrum and, hence, higher chance of survival. Moreover, last-born pigs are associated with higher stillbirth from hypoxia due to the fact they will be staying longer along the length of birth canal while the umbilical cord became detached from the placenta.

The time interval between two successive pig births ranges from 0-30 minutes, with a mean value of 15 minutes. Longer intervals are allied with higher stillbirths or newborns with lower performance that may die later. Generally, 2-3 hours is required for the overall delivery process of the entire pigs to be born. Farrowing periods that took more than 5 hours are generally considered to be problematic. Obesity, constipation and several physical stressors such as heat are reported to extend the farrowing duration in sows and risk the likelihood of survival of newborns.

The placental expulsion stage

This final stage of the farrowing process generally passes without much notice. Failure to expel the placenta, however, causes severe complications, including infections, possible lactation failure, re-breeding problems and death of the sow. Some placenta passed during delivery of the pigs is normal, but most will pass immediately after farrowing or within several hours. The placenta often slips through slatted floors into the pit area, making it difficult to tell if a sow has expelled or retained the placenta.

Farrowing pens and crates

Depending on their productive and reproductive stages, sows need a specially designed housing system that can meet the animal's needs and maintain their wellbeing as well. Accordingly, pregnant sows are often taken from houses of their pregnancy stay into compatible farrowing houses at about one week before the expected date of parturition. Moreover, following delivery, lactating sows can also stay in the farrowing pens until piglets start weaning. Hence, the period of their stay in the farrowing pens often depends up on the time required for weaning of the piglets.

The design of the farrowing or lactation pens should always consider the welfare or wellbeing of the sow and its newborns. Some of the vital welfare requirements include: the size of the pens upon which the sow will be confined; the bedding or farrowing materials required for birth; and the period of stay in the farrowing/ lactation pens.

Different types of farrowing systems/houses are available and used across different parts of the world. Indoor farrowing systems often involve housing sows individually in separate confined accommodations throughout the farrowing and lactation stages. On the other hand, the outdoor farrowing systems involve the use of individual open air pens where sows are housed individually or communal larger enclosed spaces where sows are kept in groups provided with separate sheds for individual farrowing. In the later design, some days following their birth, piglets of different sows will often mix together leading to a multi-suckling system.

Despite of the different farrowing systems in practice, the use of individual crates for farrowing and lactation are reported to be of primary choice and more advantageous to sows and the newborns as well. In individual farrowing systems, the most convenient and commonly used average area to be made for each sow is about 2.25 0.6m2, where the length can vary between 2.0-2.5m while the width is always set to 0.6m. Although there are several items to use, the flooring materials used should generally meet the wellbeing of the sow and contain suitable beddings as well. Furthermore, the flooring material should have a smaller meshed exit at the hind of the crate for easier removal of excreta and water washes of the crate. Drinking and feeding materials should further be made and placed at the frontage of the crate.

Advantages of farrowing crates over pens:

A higher record of the newly born piglets has been reported to occur before their weaning stage, and particularly in the first week of their birth. The importance of using farrowing pens and/or crates is, in general, for optimizing or maximizing the likelihood of survival of newborns. However, several research works so far done since the last three centuries have all indicated higher survival rates of piglets farrowed in crates than open pens.

Several advantages have been mentioned for using crates than pens for farrowing. The following merits are summarized for both the newly born litter and the dam as well.

Advantages of farrowing crates

- It reduces sow activity in crates, thereby reducing piglet mortality
- It increases the suckling activity of piglets
- It reduces the risk of chilling and crushing of piglets
- It reduces cross-suckling and competition among piglets for same udder of sows
- It allows maximum feed intake for each sow kept individually in the crate
- It improves feeding behavior of sows to be taken in a silence and non-energy wasting environment
- It reduces aggression behavior which is common with penned farrowing sows.
- It is easy to carry out the regular husbandry management and health care procedures. Farrowing pens often require restraining of the sow to do these activities to safeguard the risk of the working person.
- There is efficient utilization of building spaces and, hence, reduced capital

expenses when compared to pens.

Due to the fact that the behavioral, physiological, and environmental requirements of the sow and piglets are quite different, hence, maximum effort should be done for addressing their wellbeing when making farrowing crates or pens. If farrowing crates are not allowed to optimize or balance the two requirements, there will be higher chance for increased piglet mortality following parturition. Sows farrowing in crates or pens that do not fulfill their wellbeing requirements do often live the environment soon after birth leading to starvation, chilling, and reduced colostrum intake all causing higher mortality rates of piglets.

In general, the design of a contemporary farrowing and lactation crate should allow for a suitable environment to work with at time of need, and for introducing of improved husbandry and management protocols.

Care of the sow before and during farrowing

The farrowing stage of sows is among the most vital phases in swine production. A significant quantity of piglets does often occur following mismanagement during and before this period. Therefore, greater knowledge and sympathetic on the overall events and the sows behaviors that take place before and during the delivery periods are crucial for an improved care and management of the sow and, hence, the animals production and productivity as well.

16.2 Post-Farrowing Problems

Savaging

This is a condition where the sow tries to bite or kill its newborns following farrowing. This behavioral problem is more commonly seen in confined sows than pasture-farrowed ones and in obese or fatty sows. It is believed that the pain the sow is facing during the farrowing period will force the sow to react nervously and bite the first-born pigs to their death. Furthermore, sows allowed to deliver in a new or strange farrowing environment will often show such behavioral problems. Hence, the use of tranquilizers in severe farrowing cases and the removal of immediate newborns into a temporary warm-box until delivery is completed are reported to alleviate the problem. However, if sows do frequently show such a behavior, then culling is highly recommended from the herd.

Lameness

Lameness in farrowing sows could be due to several reasons. It reduces the sow's performance during lactation and reduces the size and weight of litter too. The presence of rough and slippery floorings causes injuries to the foot pads which may act as a nidus for lameness causing bacteria. Furthermore, injuries to the hind legs resulting from the delivery of larger sized litters can also result in sow lameness although it is for a short period of time. Lameness can affect the overall activity of sows reducing their nursing efficiency and may lead to stepping of the sow on the newborn pigs. Moreover, a lame sow does often rarely get up to eat and drink and this will intern cause reduced milk yield and, hence, litter performance.

Lack of appetite

Lack of appetite, sickness, hypogalactia and constipation are frequently found at the same time in the farrowing house. It is difficult to establish cause and result relationships among these four factors, since each contributes to the severity of the others. Good management, however, can generally reduce the incidence of all four conditions. Prevent constipation by using a laxative in the farrowing ration. Sows that fail to form a stool by two to three days after farrowing should receive a prescribed injectable or oral veterinary laxative or related medicaments.

Lack of appetite in the sow is a symptom of sickness and/or constipation. If the sow is sick, the rectal temperature will often be elevated from the normal 38.9 C to 39 C or 40 C shortly after farrowing. If a temperature of more than 41 C is observed, veterinary attention is advisable. Improve appetite and feed intake by using more palatable rations or cooler environmental temperatures.

Chapter 17

Lactation and Its Management in Sows

—Dr. Awot Teklu

17.1 Mammary Glands of the Sow

Once farrowing is done, the sow should then start producing and supplying milk to the newborns. The process of milk production (lactogenesis) takes place by the mammary glands within the udder of the sow. Once produced, milk comes out through the teats via small canals to be suckled by the newly born pigs.

The number, size, and placement of the teats often vary from sow to sow depending on the species, growth husbandry, and management of the sow. Such differences are often reported to result in differences in milk yield among teats, and, hence, differences in growth performance and survival rates of suckling pigs. For instance, Robert, (2009) have stated that the front pair of teats are usually more widely and symmetrically placed than the hind ones leading to a relatively higher milk production and faster growth performance of the suckling piglets.

Moreover, the competition among newborns for the best producing teats are seen to occur during the first week following their birth, and the larger and stronger pigs will be the fittest to nurse the highly productive front teats. Hence, it is highly advisable to initially search for replacement sows or gilts with higher number (12-14) of teats that are functioning or healthy, and evenly or symmetrically placed.

17.2 Milk Composition of Sows

Similar to that of the cow and ewe, the nutrient composition of the milk of sows often varies depending on the genetic makeup or species of the animal, nutrition, and the stage of lactation. However, the sow's milk generally contain a relatively lower water and higher percentage of proteins due to the fact that the first day milk (colostrum) contains higher levels of immunoglobulins, it often contains higher percentages of proteins and total solids than normal milk (table 17.1). Moreover, it has also been documented that the milk contents of lactose and fat increases and that of proteins decreases proportionally with the advancement of lactation.

Table 17.1: Percentage composition of the normal milk and colostrum of sows.

Contents	*Per cent Distribution (%)*	
	Normal milk	*Colostrum*
Total solids (TS)	20	30
Proteins	5.4	17
Lactose	5	3
Fat	8.3	7.5
Ash	0.8	0.6

(Source: Dove, 2009)

17.3 Nutrition and feeding management of sows during lactation

In addition to farrowing, the lactational stage is also a second stage requiring an attention in the sow production business. During this period, proper nutrition and feeding management of sows is highly important for a proper health and survival of the sow and newly born piglets. Despite of the presence of other influencing factors, problems related to feeding and feeding management of lactating sows are the major factors contribution to high pig mortality and poor productive and reproductive performances.

The overall objective of feeding lactating sows is in order to maintain an optimum energy and other nutrient balance during lactation and, thereby, minimize instant and/or future problems related to reproductive and productive performance of the herd. In order to successfully meet this objective, formulated diets containing optimum and economic concentrations from each of the nutrient requirements should be prepared and given for lactating sows based on standard feeding systems. In addition to the proper nutrition and feeding management, there are also other external factors that influence the feed intake of sows. Hence, an appropriate feeding program together with a concomitant understanding on the factors affecting feed intake will result in a better sow and litter performance.

Nutritionally, there should be a minimum negative nutrient balance accompanied by a maximum milk production in the nutrition program of a lactating sow. The nutrient requirements of lactating sows often varies depending on the body weight of the animal, the quantity and quality of milk yielded, and on the housing environment where the sow is kept. That is, a productive lactating sow with a high body weight needs to be well-supplied with high energy and other nutrient requirements. However, if that is not the case, the sow will start to utilize body tissue reserves to support milk production leading to body weight losses and, hence, losses in productive and reproductive performances of the sow and its litters in a short and long term periods.

17.4 Factors Affecting Feed Intake

Effort should be done to maximize the feed intake in lactating sows so as to improve the overall performance of the animal and minimize the occurrence of a negative nutrient balance. In fact, higher feed intakes during lactation do often increase blood glucose and luteinizing hormone levels leading to an increase in the number of ovarian follicles, and, hence, larger litter size for the next farrowing time. However, there are a number of biotic and abiotic factors that affect the feed intake of a lactating sow. Some of the most important factors are discussed as follows.

Stage of parity

There is a direct relation between the parity stage and feed intake of a lactating sow up to the sixth farrowing stage, with the first and second parity accounting for majority of the increase. The amount of feed consumed by the sow during lactation is not sufficient enough for milk production and daily maintenance of the animal. This is, in fact, more pronounced in sows in the first and second parity of their life. Such sows are often seen to mobilize body reserves to meet their nutrient requirements. Studies so far carried have indicated that if the extent of mobilization exceeds 15% of the lactating animals' body protein reserves, there will be a significant effect on the reproductive and productive performances of the sow and the new born litters. However, reducing the number of newborns to about 8-10 litters in nuliparous sows can improve the reproductive and growth performances of the sow and pigs in the upcoming farrow.

Protein levels of the diet

The amount of crude proteins in the diet can also affect feed consumption of the lactating sow.

Any decreases made in crude protein content of the diet of a sow in lactation is often accompanied by a decrease in feed intake leading to a gradual significant weight loss in the sow and weaning piglets as well. Furthermore, extended pregnancy rates can also be seen in sows managed under lower protein diets during lactation (Patience et al., 1995).

Form and size of diet

Grain feedstuffs with an average particle size of 700um are often recommended for an optimum reproductive performance and feed utilization efficiency of a sow in lactation. Larger particle sizes can cause ulcers of the internal epithelium of the gastro-intestinal tract. Similarly, smaller sizes or ground diets are often accompanied by feed wastages that can be minimized by pelleting.

Moreover, it has shown that lactating sows receiving wet feed are characterized by a higher feed intake (for up to 15%) than those managed under dry feed. Hence, the use of water sprinkles over dry feeds is highly recommended for an improved feed intake of a lactating sow. However, care should be given not to contaminate and spoil wet feeds.

Frequency of feeding

In general, it is postulated that lactating sows should be fed many times a day. Multiple feeding are often associated with increased feed consumption and, hence, improved reproductive and growth performances of sows and their litters respectively. Furthermore, feeding several times daily increases the chance of giving fresh feed and makes easier inspection of the lactating sow and its litters as well. Hence, it is highly recommended that lactating sows should be fed 3 to 4 times a day.

Water supply

Sows in lactation stage should often receive sufficient amount of water as their daily intake. It has been reported that a lactating sow can drink up to X liters (Change 5 gallons to liter and use it) of water per day. Reduction in the amount of water supplied can directly reduce feed consumption rate, leading to a lower performance of the sow and piglets as well (Peng et al., 2007).

Environmental conditions

Higher environmental temperatures in the lactating house do often result in reduced feed intake. This condition is more pronounced during the first and second stages of parity. Hence, it is highly recommended to maintain an optimal temperature of the lactation room, usually between 65-70oF. Alternatively, feeding lactating sows during the cooler periods of the day (e.g. late evening and at nights) can appreciably increase feed intake by up to 25% of their normal consumption.

More to the point, drafts and cooler chilled environments should also be avoided for a healthier and comfortable environment for piglets too. Likewise, provision of sufficient light for up to 8 hours period are often reported to increase feed consumption and reproductive performance of a lactating sow. However, optimum amount of light should be maintained as excess exposures might depress the animal and, hence, its appetite.

17.5 Nutrient Requirements of Lactating Sow

The nutrient requirements of lactating sows has been economically estimated and formulated by the NRC, (1998). In such a way that they can yield an optimum reproductive and growth performances of the lactating sow and newly born litters respectively. However, several factors such as differences in the animal genetics, availability and quality profile of feed in the locality may affect the normal recommendations and may cause deviations to take place from the recommended standards.

Feed ingredients

The ingredients forming the feed of lactating sows should basically contain nutrients with higher concentrations of energy and proteins (e.g. corn meal, soybean meal). However, the incorporation of feedstuffs that are rich in fiber contents (e.g. wheat bran, barely bran, hay and straws) at higher levels are often associated with reduced feed intake. Moreover, supplementary fatty diets can also be incorporated if there is a need to supply increased energy levels for the lactating sow. More importantly, fatty diets are often associated with lower heat energy losses than carbohydrates during their body assimilation process which makes them preferable sources of energy for the animal. Besides, higher levels of fats in the diet can improve litter performance and weaning weights by passing to them in the form of milkfats. However, higher fat levels (> 5%) in the diet may cause rancidity of the feed and are often not affordable in terms of their costs as well. Hence, care is needed during their incorporation in the diet for a lactating sow.

17.6 Lactation problems in sows

Lactation failure/Hypogalactia

Reduced milk production (hypogalactia) is a common phenomenon or sign often seen in lactating sows. Several biotic and abiotic factors can attribute to hypogalactia. Infectious microorganisms, nutritional deficiency, toxins of different origin, and environmental factors such as temperature and humidity stresses are among the factors reported to cause reduced milk yield. Moreover, obesity, extremely higher environmental temperatures, and feeding sows with diets not containing laxatives are among the predisposing factors that can lead to hypogalactia in sows. However, improper use of management aspects can be regarded as the fundamental cause for hypogalactia. Hypogalactia can lead to either direct or indirect piglet mortality in the farm. Hence, the identification of the case in early stages is highly important for the survival of the farrowed pigs.

The treatment measures for hypogalactia often vary depending on the causative agent. However, the aim of either of the treatment measures is to alleviate or take off any damaging factors of the mammary gland tissues and, thereby, induce milk let down for survival of pigs. Besides, efforts should be exerted not to use treatment measures that may act as stressors and induce further stress to the sow lowering milk production and/or let down.

In general, improvement of routine husbandry and health management practices can be stated as the underlying long term solutions to mitigate the occurrence of post-farrowing hypogalactia in swine production systems. Such management practices could include the use of vaccines or other methods that increase herd immunity, and others that can solve the future occurrence of lactation problems in sows.

❑❑❑

Chapter 18

Production of Pork

—Dr. Endale Balcha

Pigs are reared in farms which may be situated some distance away from the abattoir where they are slaughtered. Pigs have to be transported to the abattoir using different means of transportation. The most common mode of transport for pigs is vehicle. The unfamiliarity of the pigs to the novelty of the transport conditions, mixing of different social species, weather conditions, loading density, duration of trip and loading or unloading and associated handling during transportation influence the welfare status of pigs. Transportation of one of the most important pre-slaughter factors pigs experience. Even if it is done in the best conditions, it causes marked stress or fatigue on the pigs. The stress may be related to the transport duration, the type of vehicle, stocking density, environmental conditions, missing of pigs, hunger, thirst and fatigue of pigs.

18.1 Adverse Effects of Transport

Though transportation of pigs from farms or markets to abattoirs is inevitable, it can cause the following adverse effects to the slaughterhouse.

Carcass damages

When pigs are transported together, there is fighting among the animals. In additions, some animals will be trampled due to slippery floors and overstocking. In such cases, there will be carcass damages such as bruising, hemorrhages, skin blemishes and blood splash. The skin of the pigs and the blood vessels may accumulate excessive blood which has to be trimmed off during processing.

This problem incurs costs to the slaughterhouse as trimming parts of the carcass off will reduce meat yield and increase processing time. Trimming is important as the blemishes have poor appearance and can serve as substrates for microbial growth causing the meat to spoil earlier than the normal.

(a) Pale Soft Exudative (PSE) meat

When pigs are stressed before slaughter, an increased rate of glycolysis results, leading to rapid acidification and increased post mortem muscle temperature and may subsequently lead to PSE. Pale soft exudative meats are very important meat quality problems of the meat industry. It is caused by a combination of factors, such as stress-susceptible genes, rough handling shortly after slaughter and poor carcass chilling. If the temperature is above upper levels of normal range of 37.0-39.6 °C, it results in the development of PSE pork, especially with stress-susceptible pig breeds. The PSE conditions create conducive condition for the growth of microorganisms thereby reducing the shelf life of pork. This imposes negative economic implications to the pork industry.

PSE-like conditions are reported in acute or short term stress such as the use of electric goads, fighting among pigs just before sticking, and overcrowding in the lairage. PSE meats are unattractive and more likely to face discrimination by consumers. PSE pork looks pale, lean and has soft texture and low water holding capacity and poor functional attributes.

(b) Reduction in carcass yield

Pigs are normally deprived of food and water during transport. There can be a reduction in live weight. This may be due to the reduction in gut fill and breakdown of muscle glycogen for energy. As the duration of transport is prolonged (usually more than 55 kms), the pigs will be exposed to stress and lose their body condition. Body weight has linear relationship with dressing percentage or carcass yield.

18.2 Transportation of Pigs

Pigs are usually transported from the place where they are reared to markets or slaughtering plants. They should be moved exclusively in suitable means of transport, rendering it possible for the pigs to retain their balance and protecting them against unfavorable environmental factors. As transportation is stressful condition to pigs resulting in meat quality changes, it has to be performed with utmost care. Everything from loading of the pig at farm level to unloading at the abattoir should be done to maintain the welfare of the pigs.

Loading at the farm and off loading at the abattoir should use platforms at the same level as the trucks, permanent ramps at an angle of less than 20°, and portable ramps with a slope of less than 27°. The pigs will load more easily through gently-sloped double ramps separated by central panels with solid lateral protection. Steep ramps do not encourage the animals to leave the trucks voluntarily during unloading.

The type and design of vehicle plays an important role for the welfare of pigs during transport. To create optimal loading density to reduce motion sickness and damages, the vehicles should be have flexible equipment with barriers. The area in the interior of the vehicle should be divided to reduce social stress and avoid potential sources of danger in pigs. The style of driving and the conditions of the road surface determine that any start, acceleration, braking or turning exposes the animals to thrusting. Vibrations during transport are an important cause of stress, provoking an increase of heart rate.

In general, long-distance transportation causes greater depletion of muscular glycogen, which causes an increase in final pH (pH24), after 24 hours of slaughter and development of Dark-firm-dry meat. So, the level of stress can be reduced by limiting the length of journeys and by ensuring good conditions during transport. As much as possible, journeys should be short and direct, without any stoppages. If the vehicle stops, pigs will tend to fight. Pigs should have access to frequent drinks of water during long journeys (greater than 12 hours), particularly in hot and humid conditions.

Another measure to prevent stress during transport is ensuring sufficient loading density, which allows animals to lie down. The number of pigs per load is a parameter that influences heat stress development; more fatigue and aggressiveness, lower meat quality and a higher mortality are observed if too little space is allowed. To guarantee animal welfare during transport of pig an area of 0.4 m2 per 100 kg pig is recommended. Higher load densities (are considered unacceptable since it negatively affects the animal's health and well-being, causing higher levels of physical stress, higher mortality rates and worsening of meat quality. Pigs transported in small spaces suffer more from fatigue and exhaustion, which result in increased pH values post mortem. In addition, a risk of increased skin damage due to trampling and/or fighting would be observed when pigs are overcrowded.

Higher levels of temperature and humidity in the vehicle can affect the animal's breathing, and mortality can increase at temperatures over 25°C. Temperatures over 28°C are stressful to pigs since the heart and breathing rates are significantly quickened. As a result, the incidence of PSE carcasses may easily double during transportation in hot days. To reduce the excessive temperature and humidity in the animal compartment the vehicles should be ventilated. The best transportation temperature is between 10°C and 15°C. As lack of ventilation will cause undue stress on pigs transport vehicles should never be totally enclosed, particularly if the weather is hot. Pigs are particularly susceptible to excessive heat, poor air circulation, high humidity and respiratory stress. The advantage of free flow of air at the floor level is to facilitate removal of ammonia from the urine.

18.3 Handling of Pigs in the Lairage

Pigs are held temporarily in the lairage prior to slaughter. The lairage serves as a collection point after unloading pigs until they are slaughtered. It provides the pigs with some amount of recovery from stress during transport. Handling of pigs in the lairage is important to allow acclimation from trauma and novelty of the transport, and to produce pork of high quality, the lairage should not be a stress factor. The rest period of pigs prior to slaughter allows them to recover the physiological condition lost during transportation; muscular glycogen returns to normal level, and the animals are more likely to relax. Inadequate treatment of pigs in this stage may result in additional stress and physical pain leading to further deterioration of meat quality.

Although lairage enables animals to rest and recover from transportation stress, it can be a major source of meat quality problems. Animals may suffer from different degree of bruising and injury as a result of fighting or overcrowding. It can also act as reservoirs of infection by pathogenic bacteria. Hence longer holding should be avoided as it increases the risk of carcass contamination. Prolonging the time spent by animals in the pre-slaughter lairage increases the amount of skin damage and creates conditions for the appearance of the Dark-Firm-Dry meat (DFD) defect.

Careless and improper handling of pigs in the lairage such as the use of electrical goads, beating and exposure of animals to microbial contaminations will adversely affect the carcass and meat quality. Conditions in the lairage therefore need to be conducive to prevent infections and the animals from being stressed further after vigorous transportation but to recover from transportation stress.

The pigs should be fasted before slaughter to reduce volume of gut contents and bacteria thereby reducing the risk of contamination of the carcass during dressing. The pigs should receive their last feed on the day before slaughter.

18.4 Stunning of Pigs

Prior to slaughter, the first step in transforming the pig into edible pork involves stunning. Stunning is the process of rendering animals unconscious to avoid pain and stress during slaughter. It is performed to ensure there is enough loss of blood to cause death from lack of oxygen to the brain and with high insensitiveness to pain before humane slaughtering or slitting Stunning depends on the religious structures of slaughterhouse operations and ethical concerns of clients and legislation. Most developed countries and many developing countries have laws that require stunning before sacrifice. Stunning is based on producing insensibility by striking the animal or other means.

Sacrifice of swine is carried out by bleeding the arteries and veins of the brachiocephalic trunk that interrupts the nutrient and oxygen supply to the brain, causing death of the animal. Therefore acceptable stunning systems must guarantee quick action rendering the animal unconscious without pain, and the unconscious state must be prolonged till the animal's death.

Poor handling immediately prior to stunning or inappropriate stunning techniques lead to a higher temperature in muscle and a faster pH fall early post mortem, as well as a higher drip loss and a greater PSE-incidence than a careful handling.

A stunning can be reversible or irreversible. In the first case, pigs can recover consciousness before death; therefore, the time between stunning and bleeding is a determining factor with regard to stunning efficiency. On the contrary, irreversible stunning systems "stun" and cause death of the animal simultaneously. In this case, the objective of the sacrifice is to drain the blood from the carcass, for which time would not be critical from the animal welfare point of view. Currently, the most frequently used methods for stunning pigs are electric stunning and exposure to carbon dioxide (CO_2).

(a) CO_2 stunning

Exposure to CO_2 stimulates breathing frequency and may lead to respiratory distress At times controversies arise as to the humaneness of carbon dioxide (CO_2) stunning because insensibility is not instantaneous. It takes about 21 seconds for a pig to lose a somatosensory evoked potential. This can be explained by the loss of response by the pig's brain to a shock on the leg.

The preferred concentration of CO_2 in the stunning chamber should be 90% by volume but in any case not less than 80% by volume. The pigs should be exposed to this concentration of CO_2 for 3 minutes and sticking should be done as soon as the pigs leave the stunning chamber.

The welfare advantage of CO_2 stunning is that CO_2 systems can be designed so that lining pigs up in single file races can be eliminated. Pigs naturally resist lining up in a single file. To make handling the pigs easier, the pigs are driven to the CO_2 chamber in groups of five.

The use of the CO_2 results in a better quality meat than the electric stunning – the number of bruises is smaller and the PSE defect occurs less frequently.

(b) Electrical stunning

Electrical stunning can be achieved by passing a current (1.25 amps) across the brain of the pigs. The recommended minimum voltage is 250 volts. There are two types of electrical stunning:

- Head only where the tongs are placed across the head
- Cardiac arrest where the current is passed through both the head and heart

As the Head only stunning is reversible the pigs should be bled quickly before they regain consciousness. Cardiac arrest stunning will kill most of the pigs by stopping the heart. In both cases, electrodes must be placed in the correct position to put the brain in the current path. Placing the electrodes too far back on the neck will result in a shorter period of insensibility. Placing the head electrode of a cardiac arrest stunner too far back on the neck could result in in blinking pigs.

The time span from the moment of stunning to the beginning of bleeding determines the frequency of meat quality defects. When using the electric stunning method the time should be limited to a maximum of 20 seconds. This prevents the appearance of bruises and blood splashes and also inhibits the stress hormone from spreading over the entire body of the pig and stimulating the glycolysis processes.

18.5 Slaughter processes

- After the pigs are stunned, they will be hooked and shackled around one pastern and hoisted to a convenient height for sticking.
- Using a knife small incision is made on the skin anterior to the point of the breastbone. By pointing towards the rectum the knife will be inserted. This motion will cut the carotid artery and jugular vein providing complete bleeding. Allow it to bleed for 4-10 minutes. The blood is then washed and the dead pig dropped into the scalding vat.

- The scalding of pigs will be performed in hot water (60-64 °C). The pig will be kept in the scalding water until the hairs get pulled out easily, usually using 4-5 minutes. The scalding can be done either by immersing the pigs in the scalding water or by spraying the hot water on the pigs.
- After scalding the skin of the pigs will be scraped using mechanical scraper or blunt knife. All the dewclaws and toenails are to be removed.
- The carcass is washed with hot water and the remaining hair shaved off while the pig is on cambering table.
- Singeing is done to remove any remaining hairs, shrinks and decrease the number of adhering micro-organisms and leaves an attractive clean appearance
- Scrap and clean the pig thoroughly. Open up by making an incision on the mid-line the ventral side from the rectum to the point of the jaw
- Split the breastbone
- Loosen the bung and pull out several inches until it is free and then tie it with string
- Open the body cavity carefully to avoid cutting of guts.
- Take out intestines, liver and stomach
- Cut the diaphragm and take out lungs and heart, including the aorta.
- Remove the head at the atlas joint
- Make an incision down the median line of the back, all the way from the tail to the anterior end.
- Split down the carcass at the middle of the backbone using splitting saw.
- Wash the carcass with cold water, both outside and inside.
- Chill the carcass as rapidly as possible.
- Carcass and all visceral organs should be examined to determine whether carcass and all edible offal are fit for human consumption.

18.6 Meat Inspection

The meat or pork supplied for the market should be safe for consumers. For this thorough examination of live pigs ante mortem examination) and slaughtered pigs (postmortem) examination should be practiced. The advantages of meat inspection at pig slaughterhouses are:

- To ensure that only apparently healthy and physiologically normal pigs are slaughtered for human consumption
- To ensure that meat from slaughtered pigs is free from disease, wholesome and of no risk to human health

The above objectives can be achieved by ante mortem and postmortem inspection procedures and by hygienic dressing with minimum contamination.

Ante Mortem Inspection

Ante mortem examination of pigs helps to screen diseased animals from apparently healthy. If the ante mortem examination is not properly performed, dirty and diseased pigs shall be slaughtered undetected and increases the chance of contamination on the killing floor. The advantage of conducting ante mortem examination is to identify animals which are suspected of showing deviation from normal behavior or appearance that could render the carcass unfit for human consumption. Some abnormalities like neurological diseases of pigs can only be detected during ante mortem examination.

During ante mortem examination both sides of an animal should be examined at rest and in motion. The examination should be done within 24 hours of slaughter and repeated if slaughter has been delayed over a day. Pigs showing clinical signs of disease should be held for clinical examination and judgment. They are treated as "suspects" and should be segregated from the healthy animals. The disease and management history should be recorded and reported on an A/M inspection card prepared by the slaughterhouse.

Ante mortem inspection should be carried out in adequate lighting where the pigs can be observed both in groups and individually at rest and motion. During inspection the general behavior of pigs should be observed, as well as their cleanliness, signs of diseases and abnormalities. The following abnormalities should be checked during post mortem examination:

Abnormalities to be checked	Signs observed in abnormal pigs
Abnormalities in respiration	- Breathing pattern different from normal
Abnormalities in behavior	- walking in circles - show an abnormal gait or posture - pushing its head against a wall - charging at various objects and acting aggressively - showing a dull and anxious expression in the eyes
Abnormalities in gait	- pain in the legs, chest or abdomen
Abnormalities in posture	- tucked up abdomen
Abnormalities in structure and conformation	- stand with an extended head and stretched out feet
Abnormal discharges or protrusions from body openings	- swellings (abscesses) - enlarged joints - enlarged jaw
Abnormal color	- discharges from the nose - excessive saliva from the mouth - protruding from the rectum (prolapsed rectum) - bloody diarrhea
	- black areas
	- inflammation
	- dark blue areas on the skin

Post Mortem Inspection

As some abnormalities could disappear after some time of slaughter, postmortem examination of carcass should be carried as soon as the completion of dressing operation. All organs and carcass portions are to be correlated for inspection before their removal from the slaughterhouse. The necessary information for the scientific evaluation of pathological lesions in different parts should be collected carefully. This will help to ensure the wholesomeness of meat.

The necessary information can be collected by using the following methods

- Viewing, palpation and incision(when necessary) to determine the presence of gross lesions
- Determine if the lesions are chronic or acute. In case of acute cases, the postmortem judgment will be severe. The acute stage is manifested by inflammation of different organs or tissues, enlarged hemorrhagic lymph nodes and often by petechial hemorrhage of the mucosal and serous membranes and different organs such as heart, kidney and liver. In a chronic condition, inflammation associated with congestion is replaced by adhesions, necrotic and fibrotic tissue or abscesses
- Determine whether the condition is localized or generalized. If the condition is generalized the postmortem judgment shall be severe. In a localized condition, a lesion is restricted by the animal defense mechanisms to a certain area or organ. In case of generalizedconditions, the disease spreads to different organs of the body by way of the circulatory or lymphatic systems. The lymph nodes of the carcass should be examined if pathological lesions are generalized. Examples of generalized conditions include: generalized inflammation of lymph nodes, arthritis (inflammation of joints); lesions in liver, spleen, kidneys and heart; multiple abscess on carcass.

It is to be noted that the ante mortem and postmortem findings should be coordinated to make final judgment. In case of the following general abnormalities, the following judgments could be taken. Based on the degree of abnormality observed the following decisions can be taken:

- Approved for consumption if the no abnormality is detected or the abnormalities do not lead to any harm on public health
- Conditionally approved provided that some conditions like heating, freezing and others are fulfilled to render the organs or carcass safety
- Partially approved which applies to localized lesions by trimming off or partial removal of the affected part
- Total condemnation in cases where the problems are systemic or generalized and organs and carcass are not safe for consumption

18.7 Carcass chilling

The quality of the pork after slaughter is highly dependent on the carcass chilling process. The carcass should be sent to the chiller as quickly as possible.

This is advantageous both from technological and microbiological reasons. Chilling carcass post-mortem from 40 C to 0 C will give a shelf-life of up to three weeks, provided high standards of hygiene are observed during slaughter and dressing . A deep muscle temperature of 6–7 C should be achieved in 12 to 16 hours. Failure to bring down the internal temperature quickly will result in rapid multiplication of bacteria deep in the meat resulting in off-odors and bone-taint.

Chilling decreases the rate of post-slaughter glycolysis and limits the occurrence of meat with low water holding capacity. The effect of chilling on the occurrence of the PSE meat defect depends on the rate at which the pH value decreases. Care should be taken to avoid excessive chilling of carcasses as it may result in a cold shortening, which affects meat tenderness.

18.8 Post-slaughter Processes Affecting Pork Quality

In pork processing it is very important to select the appropriate functional additives. Such additives improve the palatability properties of processed food item and also positively affect the economic efficiency.

While freezing pork, the length of time needed to lower the temperature from 5 C to -12 C critical factor in determining the quality of pork. It affects the volume of drip loss during defreezing.

The packaging system is very important to the shelf life of the pork. For instance, vacuum packaging and Modified atmosphere packaging prolong the shelf life of processed pork.

The technique and parameter employed in thermal processing is important to determine the desired sensory profile. If our preference is to obtain optimal aroma frying is recommended, while optimal texture parameters can be obtained through roasting.

Chapter 19

Biosecurity in Swine Production

—Dr. Etsay Kebede

Biosecurity involves a number of procedures to prevent swine from any kind & sources of diseases. These procedures are used elsewhere in the world and should be applied frequently as daily exercise measures. Litters and a sounder of swine need to be located away from freely moving people, any kind of animals and objects. The end result of the biosecurity measures to prevent all groups of pigs from infectious disease causing organisms and reducing their impact. The measures to be taken include primarily planning and followed by implementation so as the risks can be lower in the effect of swine productivity. However the plan to be prepared will be based on the specific condition of the pig farm. This include its geographical location, distance from other swine farms, existing diseases epidemiology, the method of swine farm management, types of technologies adopted or used and what type of workers are employed in the farm.

The pig farm operational management components are infrastructures of the farm, size of the land to be used, inputs to be used, transportation means and people involved (owners, employees & visitors) & number of pigs to be handled at time of functionality of the farm. The action of biosecurity mainly focuses on avoidance, quarantine and administration of all biologicals and all in contact objects. The above explained ultimately increases their health and productivity of farms

19.1 Steps to Contain and Work Rules

Ranking of matters for implementation

Farms size matters which and what biosecurity measures to implement. On small farms having below 100 sows will have small number of employees at all levels. Thus to have increased health levels of litters and sounder of swine groups either you should have restocking the entire through having screened breeding stock, giving great attention on market sites and transportation, follow batch farrowing on time and age, confirm pigs from growing to finishing are away from groups of sow farrowing, apply similar breeding stocks up to 4 to 8 parities and when restocking new stock realize all old stock is out, is good to bring replacing stock from single source and consider the destocking to be applied in dry season so as to reduce burden of disease causing agents. The other means can be partial restocking of sows on periodic bases and all should have the same health conditions. Regarding bigger swine farms the biosecurity design has to follow the hazard analysis critical point. To apply this use of already existing methods, newly published peer reviewed articles and other past field experiences are necessary. Therefore in order to take action on implementation decisions the formula of:-

Correct Biosecurity Intervention value (BIV) = ((DEV*RR)/DD)-IC where:

DEV = Disease Exclusion Value per pig per year

RR = percent Risk Reduction for each intervention

DD = Degree of Difficulty (Ranking 1-10 with 10 = very difficult)

IC = Intervention Cost per pig per year (Depend on farm or industry experience)

Accordingly each causative agent and action taken can be synthetized using full quantity and partial. The decision to select these strategies should consider results BIV over zero.

Site of farm

Location of farm which is mainly nearer to other live pigs and their disposals will have higher risk for disease transmission. Extensive swine farm having a distance of at least 2 miles away from other swine farms will reduce on Arial and other means of transmission of diseases. Density of pigs (average number of pigs per 0.4 square miles) of lower than 100 pigs per 0.4 square miles has less risk compared to 1000 pigs per. Slaughter facilities of swine having lower than 0.6 miles distance to passing road have higher risk to contamination compared to as distance of more than 3 miles. Even roads which have higher density pigs transporting vehicle at lower than 55 yards from the farm of swine have higher risk on contamination too. Terrain of the site of the farm has also contribution to contamination when it is flat & with no trees compared to hilly and controlled from wind. When animals like cattle, sheep or poultry are housed at lower than 110 yards could increase the risk of biosecurity.

Physical barriers

The fence & how the barns of pig are built are also important parameters for biosecurity of swine. Any building which is open sided or is free access will have a risk to wild pigs, fox, free dogs and unknown people can enter to the swine farm and bring in many diseases such as swine fever. So the tightness of the fence and building has greater importance to keep biosecurity.

Newly introduced pigs

Any newly to be introduced or replaced pigs should come from free disease areas and exposed to quarantine for a minimum of four weeks if higher up to six weeks which is sound. This time help the pigs to adopt the environment, management practices and required measures such like vaccination can be done.

Swine products

Feeding or to make them have contact with swine meat products can predispose pigs to diseases. Thus either thoroughly cooked and known are safe pigs should not have in contact with such like products.

Visitors

Maximization of reducing of visitor's frequency to swine farms is among the means to stop disease transmission and to have healthy swine production. Equally making to change their worn cloths and shoes by preparing on farm is also supportive measure to ensure safety. Together with visitors guidelines should be prepare before visiting to be away from other pig farm at least for 24 hours and confirm with their sign on the record book of the farm. All workers & attendants of the swine farm should follow similar procedures.

Control of pests and flies

Rodents (rats and mice) are the major sources of infections such as Salmonella and swine dysentery. Insects traveling to nearly 3 Km distance can carry & transmit bacterial agents like Streptococcus which causes pig meningitis. Here therefore surrounding hygiene and integrated rodent control will help to improve biosecurity of the farm.

Transport

Different types of vehicles transporting inputs, live pigs, slaughtered pig products, feed staffs and water require all necessary watch. Vehicles loaded any input and visitors have to be well washed and cleaned before coming to the farm and need to have safe pig loading bay but allowing drivers to come to the pig building

Sources of material supplies and bedding

The supply materials include water, feed and bedding. Water provision cleanness together with their pipes and storage reduces from sources of infections like Leptospira and Salmonella on pig farms. When there are suspections, supply of chlorination water deemed to be necessary. Investigation of feed sources, contents, and storage and feed troughs required to be done frequently. Beddings should come out of any pig farms and ensured not contaminated by birds and rodents while in storage.

Isolation of sick pigs & disease surveillance

Daily disease surveillance by veterinary professionals supported by attendance of the swine farm is among the most important issues of biosecurity. This will help to identify diseases quickly and take rapid response so as to effectively control observed diseases of swine and isolate immediately sick pigs. This equally prevents the spread of diseases if sick pigs are isolated in their own specific area. Hence presence of isolating pen and assignment of specific attendants that take care of those sick animals needs prior attention.

Attendants training and obligations

It is important to develop standard protocols and procedures of that specific swine farm with the help of veterinarian and to make to be known and have an agreement by all workers. The standards clearly define all aspects of biosecurity to prevent diseases from coming or leaving and reducing the economic impact of those are observed.

Cleanness of water supply

When water is stored on tanks for water supply of swine farm need to be clean and has tight lid that control any contamination. Together with the tank & water troughs should have scheduled cleaning period that will be applied regularly in the farm. Regarding the source of the water when planned to be used from dug well testing the well usually for contamination of bacteria and others has significant advantage. Moreover if the source is surface water of any kind filtration before using requires attention. All pipe lines should be secured & when necessary washed using disinfectants

Ventilation

When pigs are kept indoor all used buildings should have enough air ventilation so as to avoid heat stress. Even more will help reduce aerosol transmission of diseases.

Supply of boots and disinfection

In any gate pens of swine farm there should be foot baths that have disinfectants and without any organic material. Every worker and visitor is required to immerse his or her boot for at least five minutes before entering to every pen. Here maintenance of the foot bath containing disinfectant should be practiced regularly.

Disposal of wastes

Any waste product of the swine farm that include dead pigs and postmortem left over have to be disposed on prepared safety tank away from pig pens either for burning or bury. The postmortem area should be away or out of the perimeter of the farm. Other wastes like manure are sources of diseases and parasites and can directly or indirectly contaminate fomites, equipment, feed and water to be used. If these are not properly applied as explained can be sources of biosecurity hazards.

Provision of notices

Before gate of the swine farm notices that contain whom to contact names, phones and even siren are required which will help the visitors can contact without entering the farm.

Therefore and generally for biosecurity of swine farm STOP and GO RULES which are:

S- Separate sick from healthy swine immediately

T- Take off or remove your shoes and clean them after travelling

O- Only known people should come nearer to your swine

P- Protect and seriously clean any equipment or tool or trucks after using anywhereand then GO from healthy to sick pigs as sick carries disease causing organisms that can be transmitted to healthy pigs.

❑❑❑

Chapter 20

Economic Benefits and Marketing in Swine Farms

—Dr. Etsay Kebede

The economic benefits of swine farms are solely dependent on knowledge, skill and attitude for marketing. To implement this appropriate daily record keeping will help to gain more benefits and facilitate marketing. This is also depends on the type of farming system which can be intensive, semi-intensive or as backyard scavengers. However in intensive and semi-intensive is easier to calculate and analyze inputs and outputs of pig farming. This includes piglets born and produced per sow and per year, piglets born alive at each birth, deaths on piglets and so on. In the world among the available meat types consumed by human pork is the major and mainly in developed countries. The byproducts of swine are many and include ham, sausage and bacon.

When past studies assessed it is indicated that a ratio of 0.9 between nonfarm and farm personal income attributable to hog production, which is much less than the county-level figure of 3.2 reported in 1999.It was also found two total jobs created in 1000 of pigs and swine farming and its size increases with time in countries like USA. This was proved as in 1992 enterprises of hog were 22% and increased in 2004 to 77%. As pigs need smaller expanse to feed and equally produces more meat compared to other animals. There are many types as product and by product. Among which although major are bacon, sausage and pork chops but there are also hog skin made like violin strings, drum heads, leather bags, footballs and runnels for cheese making, gelatin for drug capsule, ingredients for surgical suture, ingredients for matches, for industrial lubricants, glycerin for explosive and antifreeze. Moreover it is used as source of insulin for human diabetic patients and as valves in human heart surgery.

20.1 Swine Products and by Products

There are many types as product and by product. Among which although major are bacon, sausage and pork chops but there are also hog skin made like violin strings, drum heads, leather bags, footballs and runnels for cheese making, gelatin for drug capsule, ingredients for surgical suture, ingredients for matches, for industrial lubricants, glycerin for explosive and antifreeze. Moreover it is used as source of insulin for human diabetic patients and as valves in human heart surgery.

20.2 Profitability of Swine Farm and Its Economic Use

To determine the profitability of the swine farm costs and revenues need to be analyzed which are inputs and outputs respectively. The best method to calculate this is to find out the ratio between pork price and feed price. Examples are given below to analyze economic profitability:

If 70 Kg live weight of pig produces 60 of any currency; if 70 Kg dressing weight is 60 Kg Therefore I Kg dressed meat produces 60:50 which is equivalent to 1.20 currencies

If we assume 1 Kg of mixed feed costs = 0.15 then the ratio will be 1.20: 0.15 = 8.0.

As a result and general rule taking this assumptions if the ratio of price is greater than 7.5 profit can be achieved but if the ratio between 6.0-7.5 profit can only be achieved if management and technical activities are very good.

In here if the feed price rises to 0.2/Kg the ratio will be 1.20:0.2= 6 which makes this even impossible to make profit. This lastly indicates profit of swine farm is influenced by good management although profit is based on price of pork and feed.

Even cost price of fattening pig can be calculated with the following assumptions: For example if 20 Kg piglet cost is 20, and the pig grows up to 70 which the gain of body weight will be 50 Kg. Then the FCR (feed consumed per gained Kg) can fall in from 2.7- 4.5. From this if we assume the pig gains 440grams/day and FCR fall at 4. This pig will need 50:0.44= 114 days to reach the last weight of 70 Kg. This means the pig will consume 1 Kg of feed when its weight is 20 Kg and 2.5 Kg at 70 Kg of live weight. Following this the average consumption of feed per day on average is nearly 1.75 Kg x 114 days = 200 Kg. Thus the fattened pig will consume the 50 Kg gained multiplied by FCR which is 4 that makes to feed on 200 Kg of balanced ration. From here the cost of feed for fattened pig goes to 0.15/ Kg. Alternatively for pigs having live weight of 30-45 Kg require 0.20/ Kg which is more expensive. If assumed the feed price will be 0.17/ Kg the total cost will be calculated as:

Cost of piglet = 20.0

Cost of feed (200 x 0.17) = 34.0

Other costs = 5.0

Sum = 59.0.

Therefore taking the above fetching of pig of 70 Kg = 60 its profit will be 1.0/ pig. So that to make the swine farm profitable through having improved technical activities the FCR can be raised to 3.5; then the feed utilized by the pig will be 3.5 50 =175 Kg of feed; considering the average cost of feed (0.17) = 175 0.17 the feed cost will be 29.75 which give a profit of about 5 per fatter. While giving feeds of by products for the live weight above 35 Kg will produce the same result. As an example if we give 130 Kg balanced feed and the remaining 45 Kg by products from the farm the balanced feed cost will be 130 Kg 0.17 = 21.0. It is considered also some of the byproducts of 4-5 Kg will have in crude terms 1Kg of balanced feed and thus is required 45 Kg 4 = 180 Kg. Although in most cases freely are available if assumed price will be 0.02 180 Kg = 3.60. Finally the total cost will be 24.60 which is under 25. Thus there will be another 5 profit. In addition if piglets of 20 Kg can be found for 15 again profit will be 5 higher. Even if slaughtered and dressed meat is sold directly to end users profit will be maximize. When big cities are existing to sale swine products higher prices can be earned although transport cost should be considered. Supply of large quantities of pigs on specific time (greater than 20 pigs/month) will also contribute to improve profit.

Swine breeding for economic benefit contains normally in tropics sows of medium size and requires 900 Kg of balanced feed. For example when the mean price of feed is 0.15/Kg boar uses nearly 700 Kg/annum and costs 105/annum (700x0.15). And then let us find out for swine farm having 2 sows and one boar. In specified time one sow can farrow from 1-18 piglets while in tropics the average is 8-10. Mortality varies also from 10-50%. Regarding the frequency of farrowing per annum and in other areas the range is 1-2.4 times where as in tropical countries is usually 1.5-2.0. Therefore taking averages of tropical countries, considering complete ration & taking the following assumptions:

Piglets live born per litter will be 9.5%

Weaned piglets 7.5 1.6 litters per annum a healthy sow produces 12 piglets per year

Let us assume the piglet feed 26 Kg to reach live weight of 20 Kg

Costs can be measured as:

Sow feed 135.00 (900 0.15)

Piglet feed 62.40 [12 26 0.20 (simply consider higher as price of feed may increase from 0.15 to 0.20)]

Boar 105 : 2 sows = 52.50

Other costs (vaccines, housing so on) = 15.00

Total costs = 264.90: 12 piglets which is about 22 per piglet. Finally if the piglet is sold for 20 (20 12= 240) is with loss of nearly 2.00 price of each piglet. Lastly if there is a need to have profit the reduction of costs on boar has to be addressed. This can be achieved by hiring the boar to neighbor farms, increasing the number of sows to be served, replacing fatty boars, buy young boars starting from 4- 9 months to replace older and the boar can be partly fed using byproducts of the farm. On top of this the number of piglets to be produced per sow and per annum can be raised through selection and sows can be partly can be fed on cheap by products at time of their first two months pregnancy. Here it need to be clear that when changing swine farm from local to semi commercial it is not as such simple to immediately get better profit. This relayed on the technical capacity of the management. Accordingly when seen in practice at minimum level 14-16 piglets should be grown although the reality is lower while changing to semi commercial farming.

In Bangladesh in spite of religious taboo raising pigs has been used as source of income to owners and workers. As a result they secured their food security by raising them in backyard.

20.3 Marketing of swine

Marketing of pigs is the most considerable part of business on swine farming. Pork is the widely consumed meat in the world. When is taught about swine marketing producers need to have solid information on market reports so as to know whether can be profitability and when. Looking the long run market is also important in order to develop a strategy to broaden risks. On hog business and developed opportunities producers consider its production turn over. The major factors affecting hog production marketing include hog prices and mainly change on cost of feed.

On the determination of pigs market weights factors that have influence on carcass values and costs of production are important determinants. In order to know the optimum marketing weights of pigs the following parameters and costs need to be used. These are base value for live pig (the formulas to be used are: a. "Base value = Pig live weight carcass yield (%) carcass base price ($/cwt)" b." Carcass yield (%) = Hot carcass weight pig weight at the farm)"; premium value considers all price alterations and is equal to price paid minus base price and is the second to be calculated. Together with factors like feed cost: Feed cost = Feed efficiency (weight feed/weight gain) Live body weight feed cost ($/weight);gross paid (value) which is "Gross value = Base value ($/pig) + Premium value ($/pig)"; facility cost (Facility cost = days required for growth facility cost ($/pig) and margins over feed and facility costs (calculates the additional weight will not contribute any more costs of feed and facilities. Thus the weight group with incremental margin on feed and facility when it comes nearer to zero is optimum weight of pigs.

In swine farming in parallel to the slowly falling of labor and inputs the demand for local labor and purchased feed including other inputs became lower for every point of output. In Ghana it has been reported that from 2008 to 2013 prices of pork increased quickly from 115% to 120%. Along with the rate of return was 43.62% higher when scaled with the interest rate of banks. Even percentage of total feed costs reduced from 77% to 55% due to use of probiotic on brewery by products. It has been noted also the recovery of the project came after two years of investment. There are reasons why entrepreneurship increasing from time to time in developing countries in spite of known challenges. These include desire to feed on pork products, rapidly multiply, easily adaptable and produces more meat.

In Canada pork production industry was based on trade starting 1990 – 2012 at growth percentage of 77.9%, export percentage of 324.9% and import 1590.9% and finally the per capita consumption decreased -15.0%. In Australia pork is expected to increase from 360,000 tonnes in 2013/14 to 410,000 tonnes in 2019-20 which is also expected to increase in importation.

On the marketing of swine and their products the plans to be included are:

- The thinking capacity of customer in your product
- When your price is in line with the business of swine production
- There should be three marketing strategies which are "Skimming the cream, matching the competition and undercut the competition".
- You need to know the outcome of your swine production
- Selecting the best price of your products.
- After decision of your price along with prepare discount prices based on your products
- Suitability of your coupon for your customers and individual sellers
- When your products are being shipped consider transport costs
- You need to have sell terms & credit system
- You have to know your primary marketing channels
- Make people aware about your products using different systems

❏❏❏

Chapter 21

Basic Haematology, Biochemistry and Physiology of Swine

—Dr. Abrha Bsrat & Dr. Merhawit Reda

Haematology and Biochemistry analysis is very important in livestock. It helps in early identification of disease or poor growth performance, aiding clinicians and researchers in interpreting the results of tests on blood samples. Also, the assessment of these parameters can be used as a component of determining the health status of a herd. Normal haematological parameters of livestock are represented in table 21.1 while in different grades of swine, it is shown in table 21.2.

Table 21.1: Reference values for farm animals

Parameters	*Swine*	*Sheep*	*Cow*	*Rabbit*	*Guinea pig*
PCV (%)	32-50	24-45	24-48	30-50	37-48
Hgb (g/dl)	10-16	8-16	8-15	10-15	11-15
MCV (fl)	50-68	23-48	40-60	78-95	67-77
MCH (pg)	17-23	8-12	11-17	-	-
MCHC (g/dl)	30-36	31-38	30-36	27-37	30-34
WBC (×1000)	7-20	4-12	4-12	4.5-11	5-8.9
DLC (%)					
Lymphocyte	40-60	40-70	40-70	40-80	39-72
Monocyte	2-10	0-6	1-6	1-4	2-6
Eosinophils	0-10	0-10	0-4	0-4	0-5
Basophils	0-2	0-3		1-7	0-3

Adapted from: Research Animal resources (2009)

Normal range of blood volume of pig is 61-68 ml/kg while respiration rate of 12-15 / min and tidal Volume is 5–10 ml/kg.

Table 21.2: Haematological parameters in different grades of swine

	Unit	*Weaner 10-30 kg*	*Finisher 30-110 kg*	*Adult Pet Pig*
Haemoglobin	g/l	90-140	100-150	100-170
Haematocrit	l/l	0.26-0.41	0.29-0.42	0.29-0.46
Erythrocytes	x1012/l	5.3-8.0	5.7-8.3	5.1-8.0
MCV	fL	42-62	44-56	52-63
MCH	pg	14-21	15-20	18-22
MCHC	g/l	320-360	320-380	340-380
WBC	x109/l			
Leucocytes	x109/l	8.7-37.9	11.6-32.9	10.6-24.0
Lymphocytes	x109/l	2.2-16.0	3.6-18.5	3.7-14.7
Eosinophils	x109/l	0-1.8	0-2.5	0-2.4
Basophils	x109/l	0-0.5	0-0.7	0-0.5
Monocytes	x109/l	0-6	0-4.9	0-2.4
	x109/l			100-900

21.1 Serum biochemistry

Serum biochemical reference intervals play an important role in assessing animal health. However, for farm animals, the majority of reference intervals are set for adult individuals. Its reference in weaner, finisher and adult are represented in table 21.3.

Table 21.3: Serum Biochemistry in swine

	Unit mmol - mg/dl		*Weaner 10-30 kg*	Finisher 30-110 kg	Adult
gGT	IU/l				41-86
A/G	g/g		0.5-2.2	0.4-1.5	0.6-1.3
Albumin	g/l		19-39	19-42	31-43
Alk Phos	IU/l		142-891	180-813	36-272
ALT	IU/l		8-46	15-46	19-76
Amylase	IU/l		528-2616	913-4626	432-2170
Anion Gap	mmol/l				7.5-36
AST	IU/l		21-94	16-67	36-272
Bicarbonate	mmol/l				8-31
Bilirubin	μmol/l	x60	0.9-3.4	0-3.4	0-3.4
Calcium	mmol/l	x4	2.02-3.21	2.16-2.92	1.98-2.87
Chloride	mmol/l				96 – 111
Cholesterol	mmol/l	x39	1.06-3.32	1.37-3.18	1.24-2.74
CK	IU/l		81-1586	61-1251	120-10990
Conj. Bilirub	μmol/l	x60	0.9-3.4	0-1.7	0-1.7

Creatinine	μmol/l	/88	67-172	77-165	110-260
Fibrinogen	g/l				1.60-3.80
Free Bilirub	μmol/l	x60	0-3.4	0-3.4	0-3.4
Glucose	mmol/l	x18	3.5-7.4	4.0-8.1	2.9-5.9
GSHPx	IU/gHb		30-137	40-141	48-135
IgG piglet blood at 7 days	mg/ml		10 25-35 normal		
Iron	μmol/l	x5.59	3-38	39-43	9-34
LDH	mmol/l	x9			0-11
Magnesium	mmol/l				0.5-1.2
Osmolarity	mOsmol/kg				282-300
Pepsinogen	ng/ml		149-313	230-570	
Phosphorus	mmol/l	x3.1	1.46-3.45	2.25-3.44	1.49-2.76
Potassium	mmol/l	x3.9			3.5 – 4.8
Sodium	mmol/l	x2.3			132-170
Total Protein	g/l		44-74	52-83	65-90
	Unit mmol - mg/dl		*Weaner 10-30 kg*	Finisher 30-110 kg	Adult
Triglyceride	mmol/l	x89			0.2-0.5
UIBC	mmol/l	X2.8	43-96	48-101	54-99
Urea Nitrogen	mmol/l		2.90-8.89	2.57-8.57	2.10-8.50

21.2 Physiological parameters of swine

Normal temperatures, heart rates, and respiratory rates is presented in table 21.4 while those at different age of swine are presented in table 21.5.

Table 21.4: Normal Physiological parameters of livestock.

Species	*Temperature*		*Heart Rate (Beats/ Minute)*		*Respiratory Rate (Breaths/Minute)*
	°F ± 1°F	*°C ± 0.5°C*	*Average*	*Range*	
Beef Cow	101	38.3		60-70	30
Dairy Cow	101.5	38.6		60-70	30
Goat	102.3	39.1	90	70-135	12-20
Horse	100	37.8	44	23-70	12
Pig	102.5	39.2		55-86	8-18
Sheep	102.3	39.1	75	60-120	19
Rabbit	103.1	39.5	205	123-304	39
Dog	102	38.9		100-130	22
Cat	101.5	38.6	120	110-140	26

Table 21.5: Normal Physiological parameters of swine at different age.

Age/Weight	*Rectal Temperature*		*Respiratory Rate*	*Pulse Rate*
	C	*F*		*(per minutre)*
At birth	39.0	102.0	40 - 50	200 - 250
During suckling	39.2	102.5	30 - 40	80 - 110
At weaning	39.3	102.7	25 - 40	80 - 100
25 - 45 kg	39.0	102.5	30 - 40	80 - 90
45 - 90 kg	38.8	101.8	30 - 40	75 - 85
Pregnant sow	38.6	101.6	15 - 20	70 - 80
During farrowing	39.0 - 40.0	102.0 - 104.0	40 - 50	80 - 100
During lactation	39.1	102.5	20-30	70 - 80
Boar	38.6	101.5	15 - 20	70 - 80

21.3 Urine Analysis

It is an important analysis to diagnose many of the diseases that could go unnoticed and undiagnosed because they generally do not produce striking signs or symptoms like diabetes mellitus, various forms of glomerulonephritis, and chronic urinary tract infections. Colour, transparency, microscopic and chemical characteristics of urine and urinary sediments coupled with microbial culture and sensitivity test is likely to identify majority of the lower urinary tract disorders in domestic animals. Reference values for various urinary parameters in different species is presented in table 21.6.

Table-21.6. Reference values for various urinary parameters in different species.

Sr. No	*Parameters*	*Pig*	*Cattle*	*Sheep*	*Goat*	*Horse*	*Rabbit*
1.	Urine volume	10-80 ml/kg	16-50ml/kg	10-40ml/kg	10-40ml/kg	8-30ml/kg	20-350ml/kg
2.	Colour	Pale yellow – dark yellow	Pale yellow – dark brown yellow	Pale yellow-dark brown yellow	Pale yellow-dark brown yellow	ochre	red brown
3.	Transparency	Clear	clear	clear	clear	turbid	clear
4.	Odour	Aromatic	Aromatic	Aromatic	Aromatic	Aromatic	Not specific
5.	Specific gravity	1.020-1.040	1.020-1.040	1.020-1.040	1.020-1.040	1.020-1.040	1.003-1.036
6.	pH value	5.5-8.0	7.0-8.4	7.5-8.5	7.5-8.5	7.6-9.0	8.2
7.	Blood	Negative	Negative	Negative	Negative	Negative	Negative
8.	Urobilinogen	Negative-weak positive	Negative-weak positive	Negative-weak positive	Negative-weak positive	Negative-weak positive	Negative-weak positive

9.	Bilirubin	Negative	Negative	Negative	Negative	Negative	Negative
10.	Protein	Negative	Negative	Negative	Negative	Negative	Negative
11.	Nitrite	Negative	Negative	Negative	Negative	Negative	Negative
12.	Ketones	Negative	Negative	Negative	Negative	Negative	Negative
13.	Glucose	Negative	Negative	Negative	Negative	Negative	Negative
14.	Leukocytes	Negative	Negative	Negative	Negative	Negative	Negative

Chapter 22

Diseases in Swine

—Dr. Nigus Abebe

Pig production on commercial farms is largely burdened by diseases in all production categories, especially in piglets. Health and nutrition are the two major factors governing physical and economic performance of pigs from weaning to slaughter. With good nutrition and in the absence of major disease good daily live weight gain is achieved with improved feed conversion efficiency. This disease syndrome has had a prolonged and devastating impact on both the physical and economic performance. The presence of disease is associated with either weight loss or lowered rate of weight gain depending on severity plus reduced feed conversion efficiency. Energy and protein required to mount an immune response are directed away from muscle growth.

Swine are affected by a number of infectious and non-infectious agents that hamper the productivity and re-productivity of these animals. In this book, the diseases in pigs are described as following:

A. Bacterial diseases in pigs

- ***Pleuropneumonia (App):*** It is a severe and contagious respiratory disease. It may affect pigs of all age but young pigs between 2-4 months are primarily affected. This disease is caused by bacteria Actinobacillus pleuropneumoniae. The production of toxins can often cause sudden death with nasal hemorrhage.
- ***Anthrax:*** Anthrax is rare in swine characterised by acute illness, fever, respiratory distress and rapid death. It is a zoonotic disease and infected animals serve as a hazard to the handler, farm worker and veterinarian, abattoir worker and to contaminated pig products consumers. It is a bacterial disease caused by Bacillus anthracis, a large gram positive, aerobic, spore-forming, non-motile rod.

- ***Brucellosis:*** It is a bacterial disease of pigs caused by Brucella suis.In rare occasions other Brucella species (including B. abortus, B. melitensis) can infect pigs. It has negative impacts of production performance. It causes inflammation of testes and abortion. The carrier status persists during long periods of time.
- ***Atrophic Rhinitis:***Atrophic rhinitis is an infectious disease characterized by sneezing, snorting, and sometimes nosebleed which may progress to atrophy and distortion of the turbinates, nasal and facial bones of some affected pigs. The etiology is complex and involvestoxigenic strains of Bordetella bronchiseptica and Pasteurella multocida (primarily type D).
- ***Mastitis – Metritis – Agalactia (MMA) Syndrome:*** The MMA syndrome is clinically characterized by anorexia, lethargy, disinterest in the piglets, fever, swelling of the mammary glands and agalactia, and occurs in sows between 12 and 48 hours after farrowing. Escherichia coli and Klebsiella pneumonia are the causative agents.
- ***Exudative Epidermitis:*** Exudative epidermitis of sucking pigs is caused by Staphylococcus spp. like Staphylococcus hyos; S. hyicus and characterized by the appearance of an acute, generalised seborrhoeic dermatitis. It is also called as greasy pig disease because of the clinical manifestation.
- ***Erysipelas:*** Erysipelas is an infectious disease of pigs and appears in an acute, septicaemic form characterized by diamond shaped skin lesions, and a chronic form manifested by a non-suppurative arthritis and a vegetative endocarditis. It is caused by Erysipelothrix rhusiopathie (insidiosa).
- ***Colibacillosis:*** It is one of the most common diseases of new-born farm animals. It is caused by pathogenic Escherichia coli. It is of two form: enteric colibacillosis manifested by varying degrees of diarrhoea, dehydration and death in a few days if not treated and septicaemic colibacillosis manifested by septicaemia and rapid death in several hours after onset.
- ***Glasser's Disease:*** The Glässer's disease is caused by a bacteria called Haemophilus parasuis. It is also called as infectious polyarthritis. This is a fibrinous, occasionally fatal, polyserositis, pleurisy and polyarthritis of young pigs.
- ***Foot Rot:*** Foot rot an infectious disease of swine characterized by inflammation of the sensitive tissues of the feet and severe lameness and all age groups are susceptible. It is caused by Fusobacterium necrophorum, Corynebacterium pyogenes (Secondary infections after trauma). Transmission is highest where conditions are wet underfoot and in wet humid seasons.
- ***Swine Dysentery:*** This is a highly fatal disease of pigs characterized by muco-haemorrhagic diarrhoea and death if untreated for a few days. It is most common in the 7 to 16 week old age group. It is caused by Treponema hyodysenteriae.
- ***Enzootic pneumonia (EP):*** The main issue associated with Mycoplasma hyopneumoniae infections is chronic respiratory disease. This pathogen usually amplifies the severity of other infections, including flu and PRRS.

- ***Pasteurellosis:*** It is a bacterial disease (caused by Pasteurella multocida type A) thatcause of pneumonia as secondary infection to another respiratory pathogen (enzootic pneumonia, PRRS, flu). The strains are usually involved in respiratory diseases in swine.
- ***Streptococcal infections:*** Streptococcus suis is the most important streptococcus of pigs causing pneumonia, septicemia, arthritis and encephalitis in pigs and is also of great public importance for its zoonotic potential. The occurrence of this disease is worldwide. Pre-weaning piglets, weaners, growers/ finishers, and human are at risk.
- ***Botulism:*** Toxins produced by Clostridium botulinum cause a progressive flaccid paralysis, but pigs are very resistant to the toxin.
- ***Campylobacter:*** The Campylobacter infection, although it is usually subclinical, mainly affects piglets causing diarrhea.
- ***Salmonellosis:*** Salmonellosis is an important bacterial disease in swine for its capacity to produce food intoxication in humans. Clinically, Salmonellosis appears as diarrhea, systemic disease or pneumonia.
- *Tetanus:* Clostridium tetani produces toxins that affect the central nervous system causing hypersensitivity, stiffness in legs and muscles, and opisthotonos.
- ***Tuberculosis:*** Swine tuberculosis is rare today, being the most common the Mycobacterium avium complex. It causes nodules in the lymph nodes of the neck resulting in the seizure of carcasses at the slaughterhouse.

B. Viral diseases in pigs

- ***Classical Swine Fever:*** Classical swine fever is serious and often fatal viral diseases in pigs. It is a systemic disease and it is notifiable in most countries. It is highly contagious. Disease can be from per acute and acute to subacute and chronic, and can last for several weeks or even months.
- ***African swine fever:*** African swine fever (ASF) is peracute, highly infectious and fatal viral infection of pigs indistinguishable on the field from Classical Swine Fever. It is caused by a large DNA virus of the Asfarviridae family, which also infects ticks of the genus Ornithodoros. It is a systemic disease and is notifiable on most countries.
- ***Swine influenza:*** Swine influenza is a highly contagious viral infection of pigs. It is a respiratory disease of high importance due to its fast transmission and zoonotic potential. The disease in swine occurs within a herd either as an epizootic or enzootic form. Morbidity rates can reach 100% with swine influenza infections, while mortality rates are generally low.
- ***Foot-and-mouth disease:*** This is an acute, highly contagious viral disease of cloven footed animals but most important in cattle and pigs. Its occurrence is in Africa, Asia, Eastern Europe; South America and notifiable in all countries. It affects all age group of pigs characterized by lameness, blisters on tongue, snout and feet.

- ***Blue eye disease:*** This viral disease is caused by a paramyxovirus produces nervous symptoms and often produces corneal opacity (developing a blue color). This disease is unique to pigs. When it appears in a susceptible breeding farm, the first clinical signs are usually seen in the farrowing rooms.
- ***Aujeszky's disease:*** Aujeszky's disease, or pseudorabies, is a contagious viral disease that primarily affects pigs. The virus causes reproductive and severe neurological disease in affected animals; death is common. Younger animals are the most severely affected. Piglets usually have a fever, stop eating, and show neurological signs (seizures, paralysis), and often die within 24-36 hours. Older pigs may show similar symptoms, but often have respiratory signs (coughing, sneezing, difficulty breathing) and vomiting, are less likely to die and generally recover in 5-10 days.
- ***Bovine viral diarrhoea virus:*** Disease caused by two pestivirus of the same group of swine fever. In pig breeding herds it cause reproductive problems and cause poor conception rates, a few abortions, foetal death, mummification, small litters and low birth weights.
- ***Nipah virus disease:*** The Nipah virus causes a respiratory disease in pigs with a huge zoonotic consequence.
- ***The Porcine Reproductive and Respiratory Syndrome (PRRS):*** The disease also named blue ear disease. It is a widespread disease affecting domestic pigs of any age. Disease characterized by reproductive impairment or failure in breeding animals, and respiratory disease in pigs of any age.
- ***Swine vesicular disease:*** Swine vesicular disease (SVD) is a vesicular condition of pigs resulting from infection with SVD virus. Disease is clinically indistinguishable from foot-and-mouth disease (FMD) and is thus important in the differential diagnosis of the latter disease.
- ***Porcine circovirosis:*** Porcine circovirus is caused by porcine circovirus type 2 (PCV2) and has a huge economic impact. Clinically it is presented as a disease which deteriorates animals from the weaning to the finishing period producing a high mortality rate. It also causes dermatitis and nephropathia with high mortality.
- ***Swine pox:*** The disease is caused by swine pox virus, a member of the Poxviridae family that occurs worldwide. It occurs only in swine of all age groups. The disease that is characterized by round to oval cutaneous lesions that heal in three to four weeks. Transmission is usually by direct contact, rubbing or scratching on contaminated pen, bites by insects (lice and flies), cuts and scratches can also allow the entry of infection.

C. Parasitic diseases in pigs

- ***Ascariasis:*** Ascariasis is the most significant intestinal parasite worldwide as it causes great economic loss. It is caused by Ascaris suum also known as large round worm. This parasite found in small intestine causing diarrhoea and damage internal organ as liver and lungs. Lung may damage due to heavy infestation which may lead to mortality.

- ***Coccidiosis:*** Coccidia are single cell protozoan parasites which multiply in the cells lining the intestine. The occurrence of disease is worldwide and characterized by diarrhoea in suckling and recently weaned pigs and occasionally be seen in growing and finishing pigs, as well as in boars, at the time they are transported or when housed in infected barns that are continuously used.. Piglets may appear weak, dehydrated, and undersized; weight gains are depressed, and sometimes piglets die.
- ***Trichinellosis:*** It is also known as pork worm, Trichinella spiralis, Trichinella spp, Trichinosis, trichiniasis. This infection generally not show any clinical signs, but is of great zoonotic importance. The infection causes muscle cysts. These cysts are infectious and, if ingested by other animals or humans, can cause diarrhoea and abdominal pain.
- ***Cysticercosis (Cysticercus cellulosae infestation):*** Cysticercosis is caused by Taenia solium andis most common in Latin America, Southeast Asia and Africa particularly prevalent in rural areas where domestic pigs are reared in backyard and free ranging system. This infections is of public health importance. Humans are definitive hosts (humans) and are infected when they ingest Taenia solium larvae infected tissues from the pig (intermediate host). Intermediate hosts (pigs or humans) become infected when they ingest eggs that were shed in the faeces of the definitive host.
- ***Trichuriasis:*** Trichuris suis or whip worm is a parasite of the large intestine that causes diarrhoea, sometimes containing blood and mucus. Its occurrence is worldwide in growing pig leads to slow growth rate and weight loss.
- ***Cryptosporidiosis:*** Disease caused by Cryptosporidium suis are intracellular parasites which cause diarrhoea, dehydration, anorexia and weight loss.
- ***Toxoplasmosis:*** The occurrence of disease is worldwide in pigs. Disease is usually subclinical but of zoonotic importance as edible tissues of infected pigs with T. gondii when ingested as undercooked pork can become a source of infection for humans. Disease occurs through contaminated food or water.
- ***Metastrongylosis:*** Also known as lung worm infestation. The occurrence of disease is worldwide and it infects mainly pigs and wild boars. Infection may occur with any one or more of three species of metastrongyle nematodes i.e. Metastrongylus elongatus (apri), M. pudendotectusand M. salmi. Metastrongylus elongates. Pigs of any age can be infected but heavy infections occur mostly in young pigs over six weeks of age. The parasites are found in the bronchi and bronchioles and cause pneumonia.
- ***Louse infestation:*** Louse infestation in pigs occur worldwide. Haematopinus suis (louse) is of size 4-6mm usually found in ears (often in the ear canal), on the skin behind the ears, in the folds of the neck, and on the medial aspects of the legs. It is frequently present in backyard and free ranging swine farming.

- *Mange:* Scabies is a skin disease caused by an external parasite (mite) which is characterized by severe swelling that affects the growth of pigs.

D. Nutritional deficiencies in pigs

- *Energy deficiency:* Reduced growth rate, loss of body weight, birth of weak and undersized piglets, short lactation length and prolong anoestrous which ultimately affect production and reproduction.
- *Protein deficiency:* Anorexia, lowered feed intake, reduced weight gain, poor feed conversion, lack of muscle development, reduced milk production, delayed post weaning estrous and poor immunity.
- *Fat deficiency:* Hair loss, scaly dermatitis, skin necrosis on the neck and shoulders, and an unthrifty appearance in growing pigs.
- *Vitamin E/Selenium deficiency:* Deficiency symptoms are anorexia, depression with muscle weakness, lowered body temperature poor reproduction and impaired immune system. May cause sudden death in recently weaned piglets.
- *Vitamin K deficiency:* Deficiency increases blood clotting time and pig may die due to haemorrhages. Certain components in mouldy feed and excessive levels of dietary calcium interfere with vitamin K activity, causing these signs.
- *Thiamine deficiency:* Deficiency symptom include reduced appetite and body weight, vomiting, weak pulse, subnormal body temperature, nervous signs, sudden death due to heart failure.
- *Riboflavin deficiency:* Deficiency symptom include anoestrous in post pubertal gilt. Sows exhibit anorexia and farrow pre mature dead pigs. Growing pigs show anorexia, poor growth and feed efficiency, rough hair coat, dermatitis, alopecia, stiffness, unsteady gait, scours, ulcerative colitis, inflammation of anal mucosa, vomiting, cataracts, light sensitivity and decreased immune response.
- *Niacin deficiency:* Deficiency symptom include diarrhoea, weight loss, loss of appetite, weakness, rough skin and coat, dermatitis on the ears, exfoliate type dermatitis, hair loss, degeneration of nervous system.
- *Pantothenic acid deficiency:* Deficiency symptom include goose-stepping gait, ataxia, anorexia and a non-infectious bloody diarrhoea. Necrotic enteritis, ulceration and haemorrhages in the large intestine, Bloody faeces may also observed.
- *Pyridoxine deficiency:* Deficiency symptom include anorexia, decreased growth, dermatitis, diarrhoea, rough hair coat, scaly skin.
- *Choline deficiency:* Deficiency symptom include incoordination, abnormal shoulder conformation, poor conformation (short legs, pot-belly), reduced litter size and may give birth to splay legged pigs.
- *Biotin deficiency:* Deficiency symptom include excessive hair loss, dry and rough dermatitis with brown exudate, skin ulcerations and dermatitis, exudates around the eyes, inflammation of the mucous membranes of

the mouth, transverse cracking of the hooves, and cracking or bleeding of the footpads.

- ***Vitamin B12 deficiency:*** Deficiency symptom appeared in neonatal pigs fed synthetic diets low in vitamin B12 show hyperirritability, voice failure, pain and incoordination in the hindquarters.
- ***Iron and copper deficiency:*** Low haemoglobin and RBC count, pale mucous membranes, skin oedema about the neck and shoulders, listlessness, and spastic breathing (thumps). At necropsy, enlargement of the heart and spleen, hydropericardium, ascites, oedema in various tissues and fatty changes in the liver are seen.
- ***Calcium and phosphorus deficiency:*** Deficiency symptom include rickets in growing pigs and osteomalacia in mature pigs. Deformity and bending of long bones and lameness in young pigs, and fractures and posterior paralysis in older pigs. Signs are similar to deficiency of vitamin D.
- ***Iodine deficiency:*** Deficiency symptom include goitre (enlarged thyroid glands) which may not be apparently visible but can be observed at necropsy. Birth of weak or dead pigs with devoid (or less) of hair, mucinous oedema especially over enlarged foreparts of the body and oedematous tongue usually protrude from mouth.
- ***Zinc deficiency:*** Deficiency symptom include parakeratosis in growing pigs in which there is dermatitis behind and at the base of the ears, on the inner side of the legs and along the abdomen. Later, skin becomes thickened, forming pimple-like projections (appear like hog mange mite) from which serum ooze out and crust is formed.
- ***Salt (NaCl) deficiency:*** Deficiency symptom include poor growth, decreased feed intake, poor hair and skin condition and attempting to consume urine of other pigs.

E. Genetic disorders and toxicoses in pigs

- ***Aflatoxicosis:*** Aflatoxins are mycotoxins produced during periods of drought and with great importance because they are carcinogenic, cause a reduction of the synthesis of proteins that affect the growth of pigs and weakens their immune system.
- ***Ergotism:*** The toxins produced by the ergot reduce growth when are in low amounts. If present in substantial amounts, they produce limb gangrene and necrosis of tail and ears.
- ***Salt poisoning:*** Salt poisoning is common, it is related with the unavailability of water, and it affects the central nervous system.
- ***Zearalenone toxicosis:*** It is an estrogenic toxin that appears in the maize and is produced by Fusarium graminearum, which requires high levels of moisture for the propagation and production of the toxin.
- ***Atresia ani:*** Anal atresia is a congenital condition in which piglets are born without the outer hole of the rectum. These pigs have an abdomen that increases in size with age. The condition is difficult to repair and therefore these piglets must be euthanized.

- ***Congenital Tremor:*** Sporadic disease in which tremors are observed in newborn piglets. They appear from birth and with age, they are reduced.
- ***Epitheliogenesis imperfecta:*** Congenital condition in which the piglet is born deprived of skin areas. It is rare.
- ***Hernias:*** Among the many congenital abnormalities, umbilical or inguinal hernias are the most common. They are considered development defects and have a very low heritability.
- ***Osteochondrosis:*** Osteochondrosis is a non-infectious condition that causes lameness in animals of very rapid growth.
- ***Splay leg:*** This is a condition in which the new-born piglet is unable to maintain its legs together.

22.1 Vaccination in the Pigs

Vaccination is an important tool for disease control in swine herds. The goal of herd vaccination is to decrease the number of susceptible animals, reducing clinical disease and pathogen spread. Attaining the maximum protection from a vaccine depends on the timing, frequency and administration route of the vaccine (table 22.1).

Table 22.1: Vaccination schedule in the pigs.

Disease	*Age and booster dose*	*Route*	*Remark*
Swine erysipelas	6-8 weeks, repeat every 6-9 months	SC or IM depending on the vaccine	
SWINE FEVER	• 7 days old (for piglets from unvaccinated mother) • 3 - 4 weeks old (piglets from vaccinated mother) • 5-6 months after first vaccination then at annual	1 ml SC	
Foot and mouth disease	6-8 weeks, repeat every 6-9 months	1ml SC	Immunity only 4-6 months
Tetanus	4-6 weeks, 12 weeks and annual	1-2 ml SC or IM	During surgery and wound treatment

22.2 Deworming in the Pigs

Deworming is recommended for swine kept for fattening, breeding or as pets against gastro-intestinal roundworms routinely. Pigs that are kept outdoors should also be treated against lungworms. It should be done every two to six months depending on the system of rearing. Growing pigs should be dewormed at 8 wks then every 2 months until maturity. Sows and gilts should be treated 7-14 days prior to farrowing. Gilts should also be treated 7-14 days prior to breeding. Determination of the pig's approximate weight for calculation of appropriate dose can be done by using following formula.

Weight of pig in pounds (lbs) = Length (inches) X Girth (inches) / (medium) 11

Length is measured from between ears to top of tail whilst pig standing while girth is measured behind front legs. The dividing factor of 11 should be used for medium pigs but should be increased to 12 for lean pigs or decreased to 10 for fat pigs. The pig's weight in kilos can be determined by dividing the weight in pounds by 2.2.

Doramectin 10mg/ml: Intramuscular injection at a rate of 300mcg/kg (1ml per 33kg) Indicated for all gastrointestinal round worms, lungworm, lice and mites and having meat withdrawal period of 56 days. It is injected in the neck using 16-18gauge needle.

Ivermectin1%: Subcutaneous injection at a rate of 300mcg/kg (1ml per 33kg) Indicated for gastrointestinal round worms (except Trichuris) lice and mites and having meat withdrawal period of 28 days. It is injected in injected under the skin in the neck using 16-18 gauge needle.

Fenbendazole 100mg/ml: Oral preparation given at a rate of 5mg/kg (0.5ml per 10kg) divided over 7 days. Indicated for treatment of gastrointestinal round worms (except strongyloides) and lungworms and having meat withdrawal period of 3 days.

❑❑❑

Chapter 23

Common Bacterial Disease in Swine

—Dr. Nigus Abebe

Pleuropneumonia in Pigs (App)

It is a severe and contagious respiratory disease with high morbidity (may reach 50%) and mortality. It may affect pigs of all age but young pigs between 2-4 months are primarily affected. Incubation period is very short and clinical signs develop within 4–12 hr. There is severe pulmonary damage due to toxins produced by the bacteria which cause nasal haemorrhage. The recovered pig may carry organism for several months without showing signs and symptoms.

Etiology: This disease is caused by bacteria Actinobacillus pleuropneumoniae

Symptoms: Sudden death with low to high mortality. Severe respiratory distress with blood stained frothy discharge from nasal orifice. High fever (107 F) with depression and anorexia. Ears turn blue. The course of the disease varies from per-acute to chronic. Recovered pigs show persistent coughing and poor growth.

Diagnosis: Based on the farm history, clinical signs, post mortem examination and gross lesions. Serologic tests, including complement fixation and ELISA for confirmation of carriers in herd.

Treatment and Control: Treatment is difficult in per-acute cases. Antibiotic like tylosin, sulphonamides, tetracycline should be used parenterally. All in and all out management should be practiced. Before introduction of new stock in disease free herd; the history of new stock must be known and only purchased from the herds free of this disease.

Anthrax

Anthrax is rare in swinecharacterised by acute illness, fever, respiratory distress and rapid death.It is a zoonotic disease and infected animals serve as a hazard to the handler, farm worker and veterinarian, abattoir worker and to contaminated pig products consumers.The incubation period ranges from 1 to 8 days.

Etiology: It is a bacterial disease caused by Bacillus anthracis, a large gram positive, aerobic, spore-forming, non-motile rod.

Symptoms: In swine, three forms of anthrax have been observed.

(i) **Pharyngeal Form:** high fever (107 F). Cervical edema and dyspnoea are most commonly observed in pharyngeal form of anthrax. Animal shows depression, inappetence and vomition. Death may occur within 24 hours but recovered swine may remain carriers of B. anthracis.

(ii) **Intestinal Form:** This form of anthrax is severe. Vomition, bloody diarrhoea and anorexia are common. Less severe cases may recover but death follows in severely affected swine.

(iii) **Septicemic Form:** This form of anthrax is highly acute and results in death without showing signs of sickness. Young pigs may develop septicaemia more frequently than older swine but this form of anthrax is very rare in pigs. Pigs that have died from the disease may have a bloody discharge from the nose, and small ones may appear very pale and dehydrated.

Diagnosis: From clinical signs and if pig is dead then post-mortem examination shows hemorrhagic tissues, copious blood tinged tissue fluid and large red lymph nodes under the skin of the neck and in the abdomen. The post-mortem examination should be discontinued immediately. Diagnosis can also be done by smears and culture of peripheral blood sample collected aseptically.

Treatment and Control: It is possible to vaccinate although it is rare in pigs because of their natural resistance to the disease. Early treatment of infected animals is effective. The anthrax bacillus is sensitive to penicillin.Prevent access to soil or feed contaminated with spores.

Brucellosis

It is a bacterial disease of pigs with negative impacts of production performance. It causes inflammation of testes and abortion. The carrier status persists during long periods of time. Feral swine are often infected and can spread disease between regions. The bacteria can survive outside the pig during long periods of time, particularly at freezing or near freezing temperatures. The boar is the main transmission source, either by direct contact or by artificial insemination. Pigs can also get infected via the conjunctiva, nose or mouth.

Etiology: Brucella suis. In rare occasions other Brucella species (including B. abortus, B. melitensis) can infect pigs.

Symptoms: Symptoms are depending on the age and physiological status of animals. The infection in sows / boars could be subclinical. Clinical signs in includes development of bacteremia, infertility in, abnormal estrus, abortions at any stage, vaginal discharges with pus or sometimes blood, late/delayed returns to estrus, lameness and swollen / painful testicles. Moreover, in lactating piglets the disease is manifested by paralysis in hind legs.

Diagnosis: diagnosis is based on previous history and clinical manifestations. Confirmation is made by culture and PCR. Serology is used to detect sows previously exposed which are likely to have persistent infection.

Treatment and Control: The treatment is not effective and very little response to antibiotics. Depopulation of the farm particularly if there is career sate.

Atrophic Rhinitis

Atrophic rhinitis is an infectious disease characterized by sneezing, snorting, and sometimes nosebleed which may progress to atrophy and distortion of the turbinates, nasal and facial bones of some affected pigs. This condition rarely causes clinical disease in the mature animal but if the breeding female has been infected early in life it may lead to distortions of the face on maturity. The economic effects of the disease include reduced growth rate and worsened feed-conversion efficiency.

Etiology: The etiology is complex and involvestoxigenic strains of Bordetella bronchiseptica and Pasteurella multocida (primarily type D). Bordetella bronchiseptica is an aerobic, Gram-negative rod leads to non-progressive atrophic rhinitis which is mild and transient and probably does not greatly affect the animal's growth and performance. Pasteurella multocida leads to progressive atrophic rhinitis which is severe, permanent, and usually accompanied by poor growth.

Symptoms: The most common signs which include sneezing, coughing, and inflammation of the lacrimal duct appears with a serous or mucopurulent nasal discharge are observed in piglets at the early age. The lacrimal duct may occlude and obstructs the flow of tears through the infraorbital ducts and tears flow from the medial canthus of the eyes leads to dirty or discoloured hair and skin below the canthus. Some pigs may develop lateral deviation or shortening of the upper jaw, whereas others may suffer some degree of turbinate atrophy with no apparent outward distortion. Growth rate and feed conversion of the pigs are affected.

Diagnosis: The signs and lesions. Confirmation for the presence of toxigenic strains of P. multocida. Routine monitoring of turbinate atrophy.

Treatment and Control: The most common ways to control disease is chemoprophylaxis, vaccination, temporary closure of the herd to introduction of new pigs, and improved management (e.g., better ventilation and hygiene, less dusty feed).Chemoprophylaxis usually includes administration of antibacterial drugs which include sulfonamides, ceftiofur, tylosin, and tetracyclines to all sows, particularly before farrowing.

Mastitis – Metritis – Agalactia (MMA) Syndrome

The MMA syndrome is clinically characterized by anorexia, lethargy, disinterest in the piglets, fever, swelling of the mammary glands and agalactia, and occurs in sows between 12 and 48 hours after farrowing. The disease is aggravated by predisposing factors such as overfeeding during pregnancy, nutritional deficiencies, constipation, endocrine dysfunction and the stress of farrowing in total confinement in a crate.

Etiology: Escherichia coli and Klebsiella pneumonia are the causative agents.

Symptoms: The sow lies in sternal recumbency, disinterested in the piglets and unresponsive to their squealing and sucking demands. In severe cases, the milk contains flakes and pus or is watery. There is failure of the sow to suckle her piglets. Many piglets may die from starvation and hypoglycaemia.

Diagnosis: based on clinical findings, with care being taken to differentiate the condition from other specific entities that might also lead to lactation failure and causes of hypoglycaemia in piglets. Bacteriological isolation of the causative agent will be a confirmation.

Treatment and Control: Broad spectrum antimicrobials daily for at least 3 days. Most affected sows will recover within 24 to 48 hours if treated with a combination of Antimicrobials, oxytocin and corticosteroids. The piglets must be given a supply of milk and or balanced electrolytes and dextrose until the milk flow of the sow is resumed, which may take 2-4 days.

Exudative Epidermitis

Exudative epidermitis of sucking pigs is caused by Staphylococcus spp. and characterized by the appearance of an acute, generalised seborrhoeic dermatitis. It is also called as greasy pig disease because of the clinical manifestation. In severe cases, mortality can occur, as the bacteria damage the liver and kidneys. It occurs during the pre-weaning period.

Etiology: Staphylococcus hyos; S. hyicus

Symptoms: Clinical signshave three forms: In per acute form (occurs most commonly in few days old piglets), there is a sudden onset of marked cutaneous erythema, with severe pain on palpation evidenced by squealing. Anorexia, severe dehydration and weakness are present and death occurs in 24 to 48 hours. The entire skin coat appears wrinkled and reddened and is covered with greasy, gray-brown exudates which accumulate in thick clumps around the eyes, behind the ears and over the abdominal wall. In the less acute form, seen in older pigs of 3 to 10 weeks of age, the greasy exudates become thickened and brown and peel off in scabs, leaving a deep pink-coloured to normal skin surface. There is no irritation or pruritus. In the sub-acute form, the exudate dries into brown scales which are most prominent on the face, around the eyes and behind the ears.

Diagnosis: The signs and lesions. The disease resemble several skin diseases of pigs of all age groups including swine pox, skin necrosis, parakeratosis, ring worm, facial dermatitis, ulcerative granuloma, sarcoptic mange, allergic dermatoses and erysipelas. Confirmation for the presence of the causative agent is essential.

Treatment and Control: Antibiotics like cloxacillin, penicillin, novobiocin, neomycin. Improving hygiene in piglet housing is the key to preventing this condition, along with teat dipping of sows pre- and post-farrowing. It is also important to reduce the potential for skin abrasions, as this is how the infection enters the body.

Erysipelas

Erysipelas is an infectious disease of pigs and appears in an acute, septicaemic form characterized by diamond shaped skin lesions, and a chronic form manifested by a non-suppurative arthritis and a vegetative endocarditis. It is transmitted through skin abrasions and the alimentary tract mucosa by ingestion of contaminated feed. Young pigs in contact with carrier sows rapidly acquire the status of carriers and shedders.

Etiology: Erysipelothrix rhusiopathie (insidiosa)

Symptoms: Suckling pigs with acute septicaemia may die suddenly without previous manifestation of illness. Most acutely infected animals have high temperatures (40 to 420C), walk stiffly on their toes, lie on their sternums, or lie about separately rather than piling in groups. Skin discolouration may vary from erythema and purplish to urticaria (diamond-skin lesions) over all areas of the body. Untreated animals may develop chronic arthritis or vegetative valvular endocarditis.

Diagnosis: Pigs with erysipelas usually show the characteristic skin lesions and are less depressed than pigs with hog cholera or salmonellosis.

Treatment and Control: Penicillin

Colibacillosis of the Newborn

It is one of the most common diseases of new-born farm animals. There are at least two different types of the diseases: enteric colibacillosis manifested by varying degrees of diarrhoea, dehydration and death in a few days if not treated and septicaemic colibacillosis manifested by septicaemia and rapid death in several hours after onset.

Etiology: Pathogenic Escherichia coli

Symptoms: Occurs as from 12 hours of age up to several days of age with a peak incidence at 3 days of age. The first noticed sign is the faecal puddles on the floor. Usually, more than one piglet or the entire litter is affected. The faeces vary from a pasty to watery consistency and are usually yellow to brown in colour. As diarrhoea and dehydration continues, the piglets become very weak and lie in lateral recumbency. Within several hours, they appear very dehydrated and shrunken and die within 24 hours after the onset of signs.

Diagnosis: The septicaemia of the newborn cannot be distinguished from each other clinically. Mixed infections are more common than single infections. Every economically possible effort should be made to obtain an etiological diagnosis.

Treatment and Control: The prognosis is favourable if treatment is started early before significant dehydration and acidosis occur. The level of immunoglobulin also plays a great role in treatment outcomes. Parenteral fluid therapy may be indicated.

Glasser's Disease

It is also called as infectious polyarthritis. This is a fibrinous, occasionally fatal, polyserositis, pleurisy and polyarthritis of young pigs. Predisposing factors include stressors such as weaning and transportation. The diseases should be differentiated from Erysipelas, Mycoplasma arthritis and Streptococcal arthritis.

Etiology: Haemophilus parasuis, H. suis.

Symptoms: The onset is sudden with a moderate to high fever (40 to 420C), complete anorexia, an unusual, rapid, shallow dyspnoea with an anxious expression, extension of the head and mouth breathing. Animals stand up on their toes and move with a short shuffling gait. Joints become swollen and painful up on palpation. A red to blue discolouration of the skin appears near death and Animals which survive the acute stage of the disease may develop chronic arthritis. Meningitis manifested by muscle tremor, paralysis and convulsions may also occur.

Diagnosis: based on the clinical signs and lesions (The unusual combination of arthritis, fibrinous serositis and meningitis is sufficient to make a diagnosis).

Treatment and Control: Penicillin, oxytetracycline, trimethoprim-sulphadoxine.

Foot Rot

Foot rot an infectious disease of swine characterized by inflammation of the sensitive tissues of the feet and severe lameness and all age groups are susceptible. Transmission is highest where conditions are wet underfoot and in wet humid seasons.

Etiology: Fusobacterium necrophorum, Corynebacterium pyogenes (Secondary infections after trauma)

Symptoms: Sudden onset of moderate fever, lameness (usually in one limb) and drop in milk production. The typical lesion occurs in the skin at the top of the inter-digital cleft and takes the form of a fissure and the lesion has a characteristic odour.

Diagnosis: The characteristic site, nature and smell of the lesion, the pattern of the disease in the group and the season and climate are usually sufficient to indicate the presence of the disease. For confirmation, direct smears of the lesion will usually reveal the causative organisms.

Treatment and Control: Procaine penicillin, oxytetracycline, long-acting tetracycline and sodium sulphadimidine are effective and local treatments of the foot lesion are necessary for best results. The disease can be control by prevention of foot injuries and provision of a footbath containing 5 to 10% solution of formaldehyde or copper sulphate.

Swine Dysentery

This is a highly fatal disease of pigs characterized by muco-haemorrhagic diarrhoea and death if untreated for a few days. It is most common in the 7 to 16 week old age group. Morbidity rate within a group of pigs can range from 10 to 75% and if untreated, the case fatality rate can be as high as 50%. Stress due to transportation and overcrowding and build-up of faecal wastes are among the predisposing factors.

Etiology: Treponema hyodysenteriae

Symptoms: Affected pigs show moderate fever, slight depression and some reduction in appetite. The faeces are characteristic. They are only partially formed, usually of a porridge-like consistency and are passed without apparent conscious effort and splatter on contact with the pen floor. The faeces are light gray to black and on close inspection, much mucus is present and flecks of blood and epithelial casts may be seen. Affected pigs become progressively dehydrated and their abdomens appear gaunt and sunken.

Diagnosis: Based on the clinical signs, characteristics of the faeces.

Treatment and Control: Severely affected pigs should be treated initially by parenteral injection; Tiamulin through i/m, in drinking or in the feed. Other antimicrobials include Tylosin, carbadox, dimetridazole and ronidazole. Effective control of swine dysentery is dependent on elimination of the source of the organism from affected pigs, the prevention of re-infection and avoidance of the introduction of carrier animals into herds considered free of the disease.

Enzootic pneumonia (EP)

It is a chronic respiratory disease of pigs which can be associated to a dry and non-productive cough. The disease causing pathogen amplifies the severity of other infections such as flu and Porcine Reproductive and Respiratory Syndrome (PRRS). Its chronic presentation is frequent in production farms working under continuous flow. The organism grows slowly, thus the disease manifests at 7 or 12 weeks of age, and is part of the porcine respiratory disease complex. The disease has high morbidity and a low mortality, and it has a strong effect on average daily gain and feed conversion ratio. The transmission is mainly through direct contact (nose to nose). The risk of transmission decreases in the farrowing area, with the age of the sows. The increase of the clinical disease is associated to the following predisposing factors including too wide pens which do not have a good air flow; variations in temperature and deficient isolation; variable air speed, cold; high carbon dioxide and ammonia levels; high dust and bacteria levels in the air; movement of pigs, stress and mixing animals, especially of different ages.

Etiology: Mycoplasma hyopneumoniae

Symptoms: The incubation period is ranging from 2 to 8 weeks. The disease affects all ages but is not clinically frequent in animals 6 weeks or younger. Clinical symptoms include severe difficulty to breath and prolonged non-productive cough. The disease can develop chronic or acute pneumonia. Mortality varies depending on co-infections.

Diagnosis: Diagnosis is made based on clinical signs and post-mortem examinations. It might be necessary to confirm the diagnosis through one or more of the following tests: ELISA, serological tests, microscopically examination of lung stained touch preparations, immunofluorescence tests, PCR and culture and identification of Mycoplasma hyopneumoniae.

Treatment and Control: Treatment is made using antibiotics and diet medications are also indicated if there is variable growth in pigs from 10 to 20 weeks of age is present and more than 2.5% of the population needs individual treatment. Inactivated vaccines against Mycoplasma hyopneumoniae are very effective if they are administered early (before 5 weeks of age) and when the animals are not exposed to the replication of the PRRS virus.

Pasteurellosis

It is a bacterial disease thatcause of pneumonia as secondary infection to another respiratory pathogen (enzootic pneumonia, PRRS, flu). The strains are usually involved in respiratory diseases in swine. They cannot cause pneumonia on their own, but are usually opportunistic infections to the above pathogens that predispose the disease. The infections do cause significant lung damage in co-infections making it a significant pathogen of the respiratory system of swine.

Etiology: Pasteurella multocida type A

Symptoms: Clinically the diseases have two forms. The acute disease is characterized by severe acute pneumonia, high fever, nasal discharge, high mortality and accelerated breathing. Whereas the sub-acute disease is characterized by less severe pneumonia which is usually complicated with pericarditis and pleuritis, cough, nasal discharge, emaciation and increase in mortality.

Diagnosis: Based on history, clinical signs and post-mortem examinations and confirmation is based on isolation of the organism from lung samples.

Treatment and Control: Antibiotics can be used. Vaccines against Pasteurella have not been very effective in the past so controlling primary pathogens is critical in minimizing the need for antibiotic use in swine respiratory disease outbreaks.

Streptococcal infections

The occurrence of this disease is worldwide. Pre-weaning piglets, weaners, growers / finishers, and human are at risk. It is caused by bacterium Streptococcussuis. The pre disposing factors of this disease are poor hygiene, poor housing, ventilation and wounds. Affected pigs are showing nervous signs, arthritis, fever and death. It is also of great public importance for its zoonotic potential.

Etiology: Streptococcus suis is an encapsulated gram-positive coccus.

Symptoms: Affected animals cease to thrive, develop fever (40.6-41.1 C, 105-106 F), become rough-coated and may die. Enlarged, hot and painful swollen joints develop later or animals become stiff, bind or show muscular tremors ending in ataxia or death. Nervous signs such as incoordination, tremor, paralysis, paddling, opisthotonus and tetanic spasms develop in that order. Sudden death may occur in endocarditis due to streptococcal infection.

Diagnosis: Based on history, clinical signs and post-mortem examinations and confirmation is based on isolation of the organism from lung samples.

Treatment and Control: Antimicrobial for 3-5 days should be given to affected pigs. Penicillin is the drug of choice. Ampicillin, cephalosporins, amoxicillin, trimethoprim sulphonamide and other antimicrobials can also be used. Isolation of affected pigs to quiet pen and given water and food, manually if necessary.

Chapter 24

Common Viral Disease in Swine

—Dr. Abrha Bsrat &Dr. Merhawit Reda

Classical Swine Fever

This is a viral disease of pigs and it is also called as Hog Cholera, is a highly infectious pestivirus infection of pigs characterized clinically by an acute highly fatal disease and pathologically by lesions of a severe viraemia. The chronic or in apparent disease also occur, including persistent congenital infection in newborn pigs infected during fetal life. The disease has been responsible for large economic losses in the swine industry worldwide. All breeds and ages are susceptible and adults are more likely to survive an acute infection. The disease usually occurs in epidemics, often with a morbidity of 100% and a case fatality rate approaching 100% when a virulent strain of the virus infects a susceptible population. The source of virus is always an infected pig or its products and the infection is usually acquired by ingestion but inhalation is also a possible portal of entry. Direct animal to animal contact is the most important method of spread. Infected pigs shed a large amount of the virus in all normal secretions- nasal, salivary, urinary and faecal.

Etiology: The virus of the family Flaviviridae, belongs to the genus Pestiviridae

Symptoms: At the beginning of an outbreak, young pigs may die peracutely without evidence of clinical signs. In the peracute and acute disease, clinical signs usually appear 5 to 10 days after infection. Acute cases are most common. Affected pigs are depressed, do not eat and stand in a drooped position with their tails hanging. They are disinclined to move and when forced, do so with a swaying movement of the hindquarters. They tend to lie down and burrow into the bedding, often piled one on top of the other. Prior to the appearance of other signs, a high temperature (40.5 - 41.50C) is usual. Constipation followed by diarrhoea and vomiting also occur. Later, a diffuse purplish discoloration of the abdominal skin occurs. Small areas of necrosis are sometimes seen on the edges of the ears, on the tail and lips of the vulva. A degree of conjunctivitis is usual and in some pigs the eyelids are stuck together by dried, purulent exudate. Nervous signs often occur in the early stages of illness and include circling, in coordination, muscle tremor and convulsions. Death can be expected 5 to 7 days after the commencement of illness. Reproductive failure including high incidence of abortion, low litter size, mummification, stillbirth and anomalies of piglets may occur.

The chronic disease is as a result of low virulence strains of the virus. A chronic form occurs in field outbreaks and occasionally after serum-virus simultaneous vaccination. The incubation period is longer than normal and there is depression, anorexia, persistent mild fever, unthriftiness, the appearance of characteristic skin lesions including alopecia, dermatitis, blotching of the ears and a terminal, deep purple coloration of the abdominal skin. Pigs may apparently recover following a short period of illness but subsequently relapse and die if stressed.

Diagnosis: diagnosis may be made based on clinical and post mortem findings. Confirmation is by PCR, ELISA, virus isolation, fluorescent antibody techniques and agar gel precipitation test.

Treatment and Control: Hyper-immune serum is given as means of treatment. Control is made by eradication and vaccination. In areas where effective barriers to re-introduction of the disease can be established, eradication of the disease by slaughter methods is feasible and usually desirable. In contrast, in areas where the structure and economics of the pig industry require considerable within-country and across border movement of pigs, it may not be practical or economical feasible to institute a slaughter eradication programme. In these areas, control by vaccination is the approach of choice.

African Swine Fever

African swine fever (ASF) is a peracute, highly infectious and fatal viral infection of pigs indistinguishable on the field from Classical Swine Fever. It is a major threat to pig-producing countries especially in African, western European and Caribbean countries. The epidemiology of ASF is complex and varies depending on the environment, types of pig production systems, the presence/absence of competent tick vectors, human behaviour, and the presence/absence of wild pigs. Routes of transmission can include: direct contact with infected domestic or wild pigs; indirect contact, through ingestion of contaminated material (e.g. food waste, feed, or garbage); contaminated fomites, or biological vectors (soft ticks of the genus Ornithodoros) where present.

Etiology: The virus is of the genus Asfariviridae, a DNA virus.

Symptoms: clinically the diseases have different forms (acute, subacute and chronic). In the acute form, there is high morbidity and high case fatality rate and the animal dies in an acute state of shock characterized by a disseminated intravascular coagulation with multiple haemorrhages in all tissues. The incubation period varies from 5 to 15 days. A high fever (40.5 C) appears abruptly and persists without other apparent signs for about 4 days. The fever then subsides and the pig show marked cyanotic blotching of the skin (purplish skin), depression, anorexia, huddling together, disinclination to move, weakness and incoordination. Other signs may include nasal and ocular discharges, diarrhoea, vomiting, abortions and death in a few days. The subacute and chronic forms are characterised by fever, depression and lethargy. Animals recover in few weeks but remain persistently infected. Chronic cases are intermittently pyrexic and become emaciated with soft oedematous swelling over joints and mandible.

Diagnosis: This is based on clinical signs and post mortem examination. Confirmation is by fluorescent antibody techniques, PCR and ELISA.

Treatment and Control: There is no specific treatment. Control of ASF includes: slaughter affected pigs and their ticks as quickly as possible; serological surveillance of all sows and boars in every herd; improvement of sanitary conditions of housing; improved hygiene (safe disposal of manure, vehicle disinfection); veterinary control of all swine and livestock transfers; health certification of every animal used for herd replacement, and destruction of every seropositive animal.

Swine Influenza

Swine influenza is an important cause of broncho-interstitial pneumonia throughout all pig keeping areas of the world. Real problems are associated with the changing viruses that cause disease. The influenza viruses may be transmitted between humans and pigs. Swine are the sole animals known to be susceptible to influenza A viruses of human, swine and avian origin. The primary route of infection is through pig to pig contact via the nasopharyngeal route. The disease has zoonotic significance.

Etiology: The virusbelonging to the genus Orthomyxovirus, family Orthomyxoviridae.

Symptoms: The incubation period ranges from 1 to 7 days. The disease appears suddenly, with a high proportion of the herd showing fever (up to 41.50C), anorexia and severe prostration. The animal is disinclined to move or rise because of muscle stiffness and pain. Laboured, jerky breathing is accompanied by sneezing and a deep, painful cough which often occurs in paroxysms. There is congestion of the conjunctivae with a watery ocular and nasal discharge. Sometimes, there is open mouthed breathing and dyspnoea especially if the pigs are forced to move. Morbidity is usually 100% but mortality is rarely above 1%. After a course of 4 to 6 days, signs disappear rapidly depending partly on the level of colostral antibody.

Diagnosis: This is based on clinical signs. Confirmation is by haemagglutination inhibition test, ELISA, viral detection and PCR.

Treatment and Control: There is no treatment. In the absence of a specific treatment, administer antimicrobials for secondary infections; provide comfortable, well-bedded quarters, free from dust and good nursing. Vaccination and biosecurity are the measurements to be taken as controlling of the disease.

Foot and Mouth Disease (FMD)

This is an acute, highly contagious viral disease of cloven footed animals but most important in cattle and pigs. Its occurrence is in Africa, Asia, Eastern Europe;

South America and notifiable in all countries. It affects all age group of pigs. The major route of transmission of the disease is through aerosol. Other routes include contact with infective material or discharges, through carrier animals, experimentally by artificial insemination and use of FMD infected carcasses as meat scraps in pig farming.

Etiology: Apthovirus of the Picona virus group. Seven serotypes of the virus have been identified which includes: A, O, C, SAT 1, SAT 2, SAT 3 and ASIA type 1 serotype. However these serotypes further comprises a number of sub-serotypes.

Symptoms: Initial lesions are seen on the lingual mucosa which later develops into vesicles. Drooling of saliva, dullness, anorexia and pyrexia may precede the appearance of the vesicles. Vesicles extend to the nares, buccal cavity and between the hooves which result in lameness especially in pigs. Pregnant animals may abort and mortality is often high among piglets. Mammary gland involvement may lead to mastitis.

Diagnosis: History and clinical signs will give a tentative diagnosis. Virus neutralization, Agar gel precipitation and ELISA will have to be undertaken to confirm the tentative diagnosis.

Treatment and Control: There is no specific treatment. However, antibiotic therapy both systemic and topical for local lesions on the legs and oral cavity is needed to minimize secondary complications.Quarantine and vaccination should be in place. In FMD free counties, infected animals are slaughtered and carcasses burnt or buried with Calcium oxide and whole premises decontaminated.

Blue Eye Disease

Blue eye disease is a viral disease that characterized clinically by central nervous system abnormalities and corneal opacity that develops a bluish color. This disease is unique to pigs. When it appears in a susceptible breeding farm, the first clinical signs are usually seen in the farrowing rooms.

Etiology: Paramyxovirus

Symptoms: It includes some animals particularly sows have bluish eyes; increase in the rate of returns, which lasts about six months; there may be abortions and stillbirths. Up to 40% of boars have testicular enlargement; usually unilateral, followed by shrinkage and loss of fertility. Whereas lactating pigletshave a hunched posture, and show coarse hair for a short time. They may develop acute neurological symptoms which are manifested by difficulty in walking, they begin to tremble and sit in abnormal postures. Some are lying on their side, making rowing motions with their legs and they move their eyeballs from side to side. Some piglets have watery eyes and their eyelids become swollen and sticky.

Diagnosis: Diagnosis can be made based on clinical signs. Confirm diagnosis by serological tests, isolation of virus from brain tissue and histopathologic lesions especially in the brain are highly suggestive.

Treatment and Control: There is no effective treatment. Animals should be replaced from negative farms.

Aujeszky's disease

Aujeszky's disease, or pseudorabies, is a contagious viral disease that primarily affects pigs. The virus causes reproductive and severe neurological disease in affected animals; death is common. It affects all age group but younger animals are the most severely affected. Piglets usually have a fever, stop eating, and show neurological signs (seizures, paralysis), and often die within 24-36 hours. Older pigs may show similar symptoms, but often have respiratory signs (coughing, sneezing, difficulty breathing) and vomiting, are less likely to die and generally recover in 5-10 days.

Etiology: It is caused by herpes virus, Suid herpesvirus 1 (SHV).

Symptoms: In sows, it causes fever, coughing, nervous symptoms, reproductive failure which cause abortions, still birth, mummified piglets and birth of weak litters. In Piglets, nervous signs like incoordination, sneezing, coughing and high mortality is observed. Among weaners and growers, it shows fever, coughing, sneezing and pneumonia, nervous signs like incoordination. Mortality is usually low in weaners and growers.

Diagnosis: Diagnosis can be made based on clinical signs. Laboratory tests like Fluorescent antibody tests, virus isolation and serological tests are required to confirm the diagnosis.

Treatment and Control: There is no effective treatment. Antibiotic administration to control secondary bacteria in a new outbreak could be done with 600-800g of oxytetacycline in the breeding ration for 3-4 weeks.

Bovine viral diarrhea virus

Swine can be infected by the bovine viral diarrhea virus (BVDV) under natural conditions. These infections are causing major economic and production losses worldwide. These viruses mainly affect cattle and sheep, but can enter into reproductive swine farms causing problems.

Etiology: It is caused by the genus Pestivirus.

Symptoms: In pig breeding herds it cause reproductive problems and cause poor conception rates, a few abortions, fetal death, mummification, small litters and low birth weights.

Diagnosis: Diagnosis can be made by laboratory tests like virus isolation and serological tests.

Treatment and Control: No effective treatment and the infections are self-eliminating.

Nipah virus disease

This disease is of zoonotic importance and causes respiratory and occasionally nervous signs in pigs. It is an emerging infectious disease which first appeared in domestic pigs in Malaysia and Singapore in 1998 and 1999. Fruit bat is the reservoir and the virus is present in bat urine, bat feces, saliva, and birthing fluids.

Etiology: It is caused by the Nipah virus which is a member of the family Paramyxoviridae, genus Henipavirus.

Symptoms: Affected pigs show respiratory and nervous systems. It is a highly contagious disease in pigs. The clinical signs vary with age and the individual animal's response to the virus. Mortality is low except in piglets. Higher morbidity in all age groups. The affected pigs develop a fever, coughing and difficulty breathing. Nervous signs may also develop which includes twitching, trembling, muscle fasciculation, spasms, muscle weakness, convulsions, and death. Some animals, however, remain asymptomatic.

Diagnosis: Difficult to diagnose based on clinical signs alone. Diagnosis can be made by laboratory tests like virus isolation and real time polymerase chain reaction (RT-PCR).

Treatment and Control: The drug ribavirin has been shown to be effective against the viruses in vitro. Treatment is limited to supportive care.

Porcine Reproductive and Respiratory Syndrome (PRRS)

The disease also named blue ear disease. It is a widespread disease affecting domestic pigs of any age. Disease characterized by reproductive impairment or failure in breeding animals, and respiratory disease in pigs of any age.

Etiology: It is caused by the PRRS virus of the genus Arterivirus, classified in the virus family, Arteriviridae.

Symptoms: Signs and symptoms are influenced by virulence of the virus, age group affected, secondary infection if any, and herd size and management practices. The disease characterized by reproductive failure in sows, and respiratory disease in young pigs. The reproductive failure is characterised by infertility, abortions, stillbirths, or the birth of weak piglets that often die soon after birth from respiratory disease and secondary infections. Among young pigs, the symptoms are fever, depression, stunting due to systemic disease, and pneumonia. Sneezing, fever and lethargy are followed by expiratory dyspnoea.

Diagnosis: Clinical signs and post mortem examination. Diagnosis can be made by laboratory tests like virus isolation and serological tests.

Treatment and Control: A vaccine exists and is effective. Commercial vaccines, both modified live and killed, have been used. Antibiotic treatment should be given for three to four weeks to all sows and boars immediately the disease is diagnosed or suspected. Immediate treatment usually reduces abortions, stillbirths, mummified pigs and early farrowing caused by secondary bacterial infection.

Swine vesicular disease

Swine vesicular disease (SVD) is a vesicular condition of pigs resulting from infection with SVD virus. Disease is clinically indistinguishable from foot-and-mouth disease (FMD) and is thus important in the differential diagnosis of the latter disease.

Etiology: It is caused by swine vesicular disease virus (SVDV) is classified as a pig enterovirus, in the family Picornaviridae.

Symptoms: Sudden lameness. Outbreak affecting a high proportion of herd. Disease characterized by similar clinical signs as FMD i.e. vesicles in face, tongue and hooves are present.

Diagnosis: Clinical signs. Diagnosis can be made by laboratory tests like virus isolation and serological tests.

Treatment and Control: Vaccination and symptomatic treatment.

Swine pox

Swine pox occurs worldwide and it occurs only in swine of all age groups. The disease that is characterized by round to oval cutaneous lesions that heal in three to four weeks.Transmission is usually by direct contact, rubbing or scratching on contaminated pen, bites by insects (lice and flies), cuts and scratches can also allow the entry of infection.

Etiology: It is caused by by swine pox virus, a member of the Poxviridae family.

Symptoms: The incubation period of disease is 3-6 days. The lesion may appear with mild fever. Small circular red 1 cm spots present on the ventral abdomen with a vesicle containing straw-coloured fluid in the centre. Lesion may be seen on along the flanks, abdomens, occasionally the ears, edge of the tongue, lips and all over the body. Later, form vesicle which ruptures and scan is formed which turns black. Anorexia, depression may be observed. Affected pigs appear hairy.

Diagnosis: Clinical signs by identifying lesions. Diagnosis can be made by laboratory tests like virus isolation and serological tests.

Treatment and Control: Disease can be controlled by use of insecticide to eliminate lice and flies which transmit the disease. Cleaning and disinfection of pen is also important as virus may persist for long time in farm premises.

❑❑❑

Chapter 25

Common Parasitic Disease in Swine

—Dr. Abrha Bsrat & Dr. Etsay Kebede

Ascariasis

Ascariasis is the most significant intestinal parasite worldwide as it causes great economic loss. It is caused by Ascaris suum also known as large round worm. This parasite found in small intestine causing diarrhoea and damage internal organ as liver and lungs. Lung may damage due to heavy infestation which may lead to mortality.

Etiology: It is caused by roundworm Ascaris suum.

Life cycle: Adult Ascaris summ live in the small intestine of pigs and it lays a great number of eggs which has thick wall hence resistant to adverse environments. Egg may survive in favourable condition up to 5 years. When eggs ingested by a host, it become infective within a week and larvae are released in the small intestine. These larvae migrate across the intestinal wall and portal vein to reach liver within 24 hours of being swallowed. From liver, larvae comes to lungs through blood stream. Larvae damage the lungs and liver during migration and sometimes the kidneys. Larvae reach the pharynx through the bronchi and trachea, after they are swallowed by the host, they mature in the intestine and lay eggs (figure 25.1).

Symptoms: Reduction the growth rate of young pigs. In growing pigs, weight gain failure, rough hair coat, pendulous abdomen, persistent coughing and dyspnoea are common symptoms. In heavy infestation, it may cause mechanical obstruction of the intestine. White spots (also called milk spots), haemorrhage and fibrosis is observed due to larval migration through liver and these signs are visible after one week of infection and it regress after 2-4 weeks. Pulmonary edema, influenza and endemic pneumonia also visible in heavy infection. Difficult and abdominal breathing (thumps) are also observed.

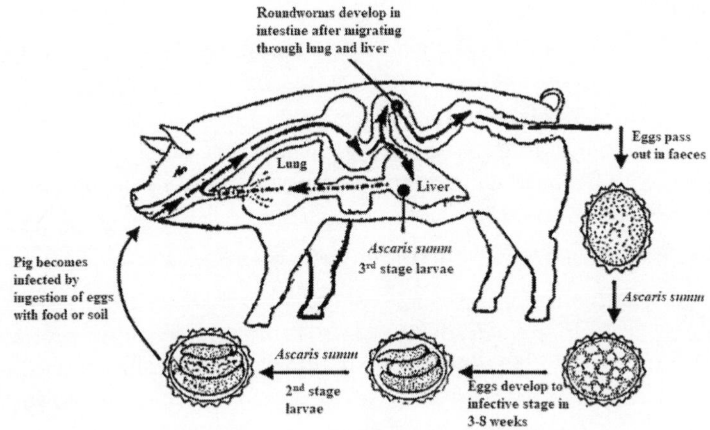

Figure 25.1: Life cycle of Ascaris summ

Diagnosis: Diagnosis can be made based on ante-mortem and post mortem findings. Chronic infestation (more than two months) diagnosis can be done by identifying eggs using fecal flotation examinations or by finding grossly visible ascarids in the small intestine.

Treatment and Control: Anthelmintics and sanitary measures.

Coccidiosis

The occurrence of disease is worldwide and characterized by diarrhoea in suckling and recently weaned pigs and occasionally be seen in growing and finishing pigs, as well as in boars, at the time they are transported or when housed in infected barns that are continuously used.. Piglets may appear weak, dehydrated, and undersized; weight gains are depressed, and sometimes piglets die.

Etiology: Coccidia are single cell protozoan parasites which multiply in the cells lining the intestine. The parasite multiply inside the host cells, mainly from the digestive tract. There are three types: Eimeria, Isospora and Cryptosporidium. Isospora suis is the most pathogenic of the three coccidia species.

Symptoms: Symptoms appears as early as five days after birth but are more commonly seen in piglets from one to three weeks old. It causes malabsorption, diarrhoea, loss of condition and some deaths. The faeces of affected piglets may be whitish and firm, there may be transient pasty diarrhoea or profuse yellowish, watery diarrhoea. Piglets usually continue to nurse but may vomit milk. Morbidity is high but mortality is variable, often moderate.

Diagnosis: Diagnosis can be made by identifying the coccidia in histologic sections. Diagnosis by fecal examinations may be possible.

Treatment and Control: Amprolium premix, monensin sodium or sulfadimidine. These antibiotics must be administered when the sows enters the farrowing area and through all the lactation. Inject each litter with long lasting sulphonamide at 6 days of age. One dosage of 6.25 mg/kg of toltrazuril controls the disease effectively.

Trichinosis

It is also known as pork worm, Trichinella spiralis, Trichinella spp, Trichinosis, trichiniasis. This infection generally not show any clinical signs, but is of great zoonotic importance. The infection causes muscle cysts. These cysts are infectious and, if ingested by other animals or humans, can cause diarrhoea and abdominal pain. The disease in humans can progress and be very painful causing symptoms of the central nervous system.

Etiology: It is caused by a nematode worm Trichinella spiralis.

Life cycle: Trichinella spiralis is a nematode which parasitizes pigs, dogs, cats, mice, wild boar and other carnivorous game, humans and other mammals. Wild animals and swine are the reservoirs of trichinosis. By ingesting T. spiralis larvae infected pork in garbage or dead infected rat, swine or other wild carnivore get infected (figure 25.2, 25.3 and 25.4). Other species (sylvatic) trichinella in wildlife can cause disease in humans.

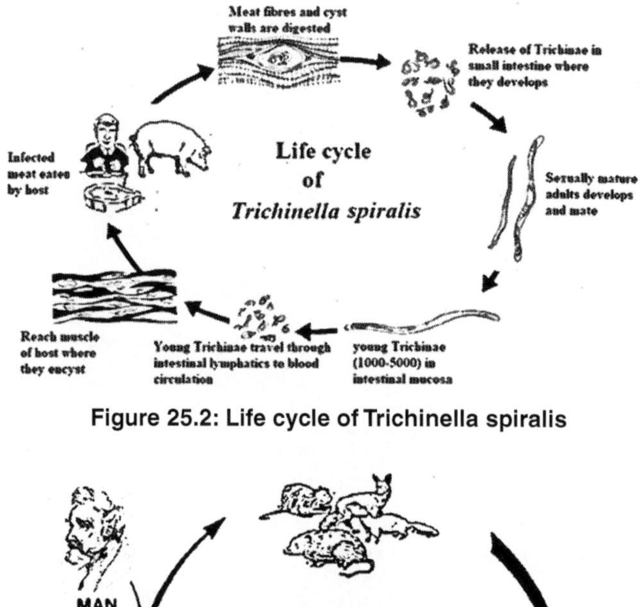

Figure 25.2: Life cycle of Trichinella spiralis

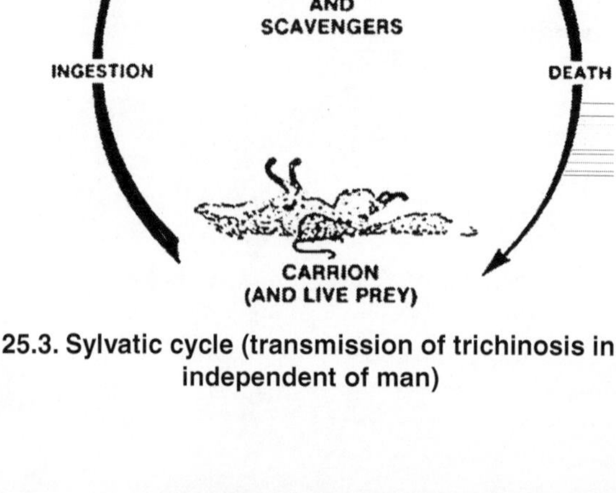

Figure 25.3. Sylvatic cycle (transmission of trichinosis in nature, independent of man)

After penetrating the epithelial lining of the small intestine, larvae undergo four moults and become sexually mature adults. Then new born larvae pass to the striated muscles where they grow, curl up in a spiral coil and are encysted.

After growth (up to 0.5-1mm) they appear as oval nodules and are visible to the naked eye. The sites of predilection for these larvae are the tongue, diaphragm, eye, masticatory and intercostal muscles. Larvae may die or mineralized when they stay for a long period of time in muscle. Swine, humans and carnivores become infected from eating infected pork, horse, seal or other meat. Larvae may survive for a long time in decaying and putrefying muscle and carrion.

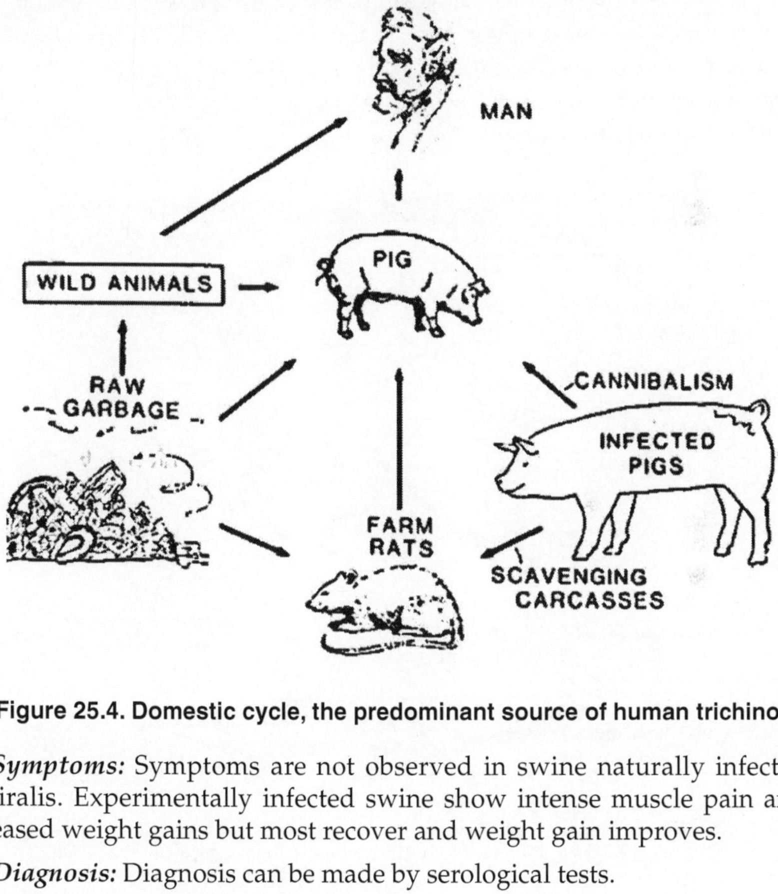

Figure 25.4. Domestic cycle, the predominant source of human trichinosis.

Symptoms: Symptoms are not observed in swine naturally infected with T. spiralis. Experimentally infected swine show intense muscle pain and have decreased weight gains but most recover and weight gain improves.

Diagnosis: Diagnosis can be made by serological tests.

Treatment and Control: No treatment for affected animals. It can be prevented by consumption of infected meat or garbage.

Cysticercosis (Cysticercus cellulosae infestation)

Porcine Cysticercosis is caused by Taenia solium andis most common in Latin America, Southeast Asia and Africa particularly prevalent in rural areas where domestic pigs are reared in backyard and free ranging system. This infections is of public health importance. Humans are definitive hosts (humans) and are infected when they ingest Taenia solium larvae infected tissues from the pig (intermediate host). Intermediate hosts (pigs or humans) become infected when they ingest eggs that were shed in the faeces of the definitive host (figure 25.5).

Etiology: It is caused by tapeworm Taenia solium.

Symptoms: It is usually characterized by mild and non-specific symptoms. Abdominal pain, nausea, diarrhoea or constipation may arise when the tapeworms become fully developed in the intestine. Cysticerci in pigs are found in the brain, liver, heart and skeletal muscles. They cause an inflammatory response in the muscle and central nervous system. In human, generally symptoms are not visible unless larvae reach the central nervous system. The symptoms of neurocysticercosis in human depends on the number, size, stage, and location of the pathological changes as well as the host's immune response. The major symptoms include chronic headaches, blindness, seizures, hydrocephalus, meningitis, dementia, and symptoms and can be fatal.

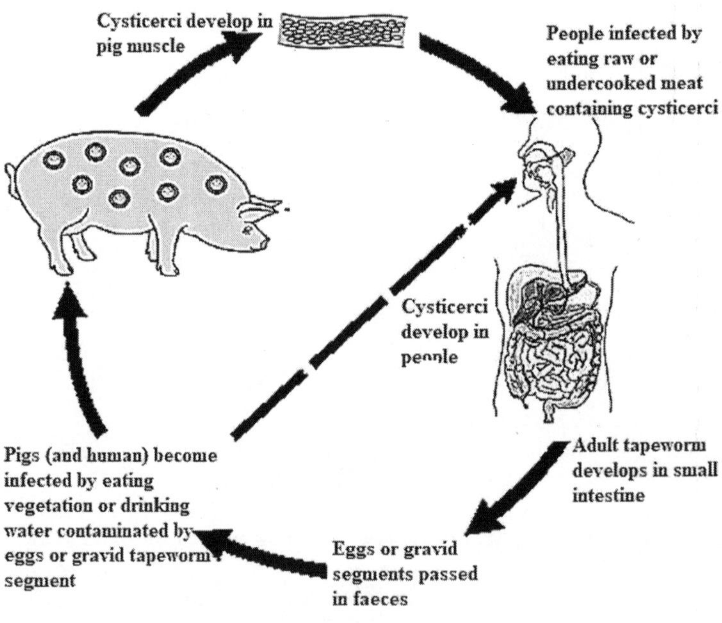

Figure 25.5: Life cycle of Taenia solium.

Diagnosis: Diagnosis can be made by ante-mortem and post mortem examination.

Treatment and Control: Praziquantel or niclosamide can be used.

Trichuriasis

Trichuris suis or whip worm is a parasite of the large intestine that causes diarrhoea, sometimes containing blood and mucus. Its occurrence is worldwide in growing pig leads to slow growth rate and weight loss.

Symptoms: It is characterized by diarrhoea with blood with or without mucus which leads to dehydration slow growth and weight loss. Pigs appear hairy.

Diagnosis: Diagnosis can be made by worm isolation in the large intestine during post mortem examination and analysis of faeces for eggs.

Treatment and Control: Use of specific anthelmintic as not every anthelmintic is effective against this worm.

Cryptosporidiosis

Disease caused by Cryptosporidium suis are intracellular parasites which cause diarrhoea, dehydration, anorexia and weight loss.

Etiology: It is caused by a nematode worm Cryptosporidium suis.

Symptoms: Usually asymptomatic in adults but in nursing piglets it is characterized by diarrhoea with blood with or without mucus which leads to dehydration slow growth and weight loss. Pigs appear hairy.

Diagnosis: Diagnosis can be made by faecal laboratory analysis.

Treatment and Control: No recognized treatment.

Toxoplasmosis

The occurrence of disease is worldwide in pigs. Disease is usually subclinical but of zoonotic importance as edible tissues of infected pigs with T. gondii when ingested as undercooked pork can become a source of infection for humans. Disease occurs through contaminated food or water.

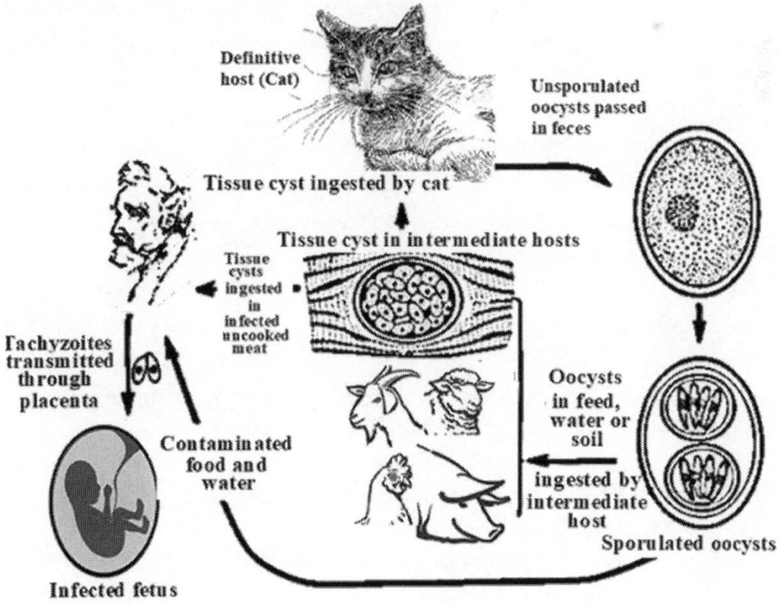

Figure 25.6: Life cycle of Toxoplasma gondii.

Etiology: It is caused by a protozoan parasite Toxoplasma gondii.

Life cycle: Members of family Felidae (domestic cats and their relatives) are the only definitive hosts. Cat shed unsporulated oocysts in faeces which sporulate in the environment and become infective (figure 25.6). Birds and rodents are intermediate hosts become infected after ingesting soil, water or plant material contaminated with oocysts. Further, oocysts develops into tachyzoites after ingestion which localize in neural and muscle tissue and develop into tissue cyst bradyzoites. Human become infected with tissue cysts after ingestion of sporulated oocysts in the environment from birds and rodents. There are three infectious stages of the parasite T. gondii; tachyzoites; bradyzoites (found in tissue cysts) and oocysts. Disease can be transmitted vertically from mother to foetus and cause birth defects and spontaneous abortion.

Symptoms: Infected sows shows reproductive failure, abortion or still birth. Laboured respiration, fever, general weakness, diarrhoea and nervous signs also visible. In utero infected pig shows diarrhoea, lack of coordination, seizures, coughing and weak piglets with difficulty in moving.

Diagnosis: Diagnosis can be made by serological tests and histological analysis of tissues.

Treatment and Control: No effective treatment.

Metastrongylosis

Also known as lung worm infestation. The occurrence of disease is worldwide and it infects mainly pigs and wild boars. Infection may occur with any one or more of three species of metastrongyle nematodes i.e. Metastrongylus elongatus (apri), M. pudendotectusand M. salmi. Metastrongylus elongates. Pigs of any age can be infected but heavy infections occur mostly in young pigs over six weeks of age. The parasites are found in the bronchi and bronchioles and cause pneumonia.

Etiology: It is caused by one or more of three species of metastrongyle nematodes i.e. Metastrongylus elongatus (apri), M. pudendotectusand M. salmi. Metastrongylus elongates.

Symptoms: Chronic and sometimes paroxysmal coughing. Pneumonic pig shows dyspnea and abdominal respiration (thumping). Other symptoms are tremors, slow growth and weight loss.

Diagnosis: Diagnosis can be done by faecal analysis for eggs and evaluation of lung tissue.

Treatment and Control: Using an effective anthelmintic on sows prior to farrowing and then moving them to clean pasture is helpful.

Louse infestation

Louse infestation in pigs occur worldwide. Haematopinus suis(louse) is of size 4-6mm usually found in ears (often in the ear canal), on the skin behind the ears, in the folds of the neck, and on the medial aspects of the legs. It is frequently present in backyard and free ranging swine farming.

Etiology: It is caused by Haematopinus suis.

Symptoms: Severe anaemia, red skin lesion and skin irritation which leads to persistent rubbing and scratching. Finally, patchy alopecia and pallor are signs of pediculosis are seen.

Diagnosis: Diagnosis can be done by clinical examination. Louse are large and easily visualized especially on the neck, flank, and inner parts of the legs.

Treatment and Control: Susceptible to many insecticides. Injectable ivermectins are also effective.

Mange

The occurrence of mange is worldwide and it affects pigs of all age especially sows and boars. A parasitic disease of the skin caused by the sarcoptic mange mite and often cause scratching, rubbing, red spots, scabs and thickened skin, dirty or blood-blistered ears, reduced growth. Marked pruritis and papules.

Etiology: It is caused by mite Sarcoptes scabiei varsuis.

Symptoms: The most common signs are frequent rubbing and scratching which is more pronounced when the skin is warmed by the sun, presumably the result of increased activity of mites.Decreased rate of growth, inefficient use of feed and decrease productivity are common symptoms. Shaking of ears and scratching of body against the wall due to itiching. In chronic cases, thick, asbestos-like lesions appear on the ears, both sides of the neck, the elbows, the front of the hock and the dorsal part of the neck. Morbidity is high but mortality from mange alone is unusual.

Diagnosis: Diagnosis can be confirmed by demonstrating the presence of the mite in skin scrapings. There is also an ELISA test available to perform blood tests, although its use is not common.

Treatment and Control: Two consecutive doses of an injectable avermectin, 14 days apart, are effective. Doramectin and phosmet may also be used.

❑❑❑

Chapter 26

Nutritional Deficiencies in Swine

—Dr. Kiros Abebe & Mr.Hailay Kidanu

26.1 Energy and Protein Deficiency

Energy and protein are required by pig for different body function. Energy is required for maintenance, production and reproduction while protein is needed for body tissue formation. Its requirement depends on age and body weight of animals and they are essential for general health of pig (table 26.1).

Symptoms of energy deficiency: Reduced growth rate, loss of body weight, birth of weak and undersized piglets, short lactation length and prolong anoestrous which ultimately affect production and reproduction.

Symptoms of Protein deficiency: Anorexia, lowered feed intake, reduced weight gain, poor feed conversion, lack of muscle development, reduced milk production, delayed post weaning estrous and poor immunity.

26.2 Fat Deficiency

The essential fatty acids like linoleic and linolenic acid are essential for swine. These fatty acids are substrates for the endogenous synthesis of other fatty acids that are needed for many physiologic processes. They are required for maintaining the integrity of skin and cell membranes and synthesizing prostaglandins and leukotrienes. Deficiency of linoleic acid leads to hair loss, scaly dermatitis, skin necrosis on the neck and shoulders, and an unthrifty appearance in growing pigs.

Table 26.1: Clinical Signs of energy, protein and essential fatty acid deficiencies in swine.

Nutrient	*Energy*	*Protein level*	*Protein Quality (essential amino acids)*	*Essential Fatty Acids*
Deficiency Sign				
Slow growth	√		√	√
Reduced appetite		√	√	√
Poor hair and skin conditions		√	√	√
Lameness				
Diarrhoea				
Impaired reproduction	√	√		
Offspring dead or weak		√		
Weakened bone structure				
Other	Reduced fatness in proportion to body weight	Anaemia Poor feed efficiency; overfat carcass	Poor feed efficiency; overfat carcass	Loss of hair; scaly, dandruff like dermatitis, especially of feet and tail

Source: Adapted from Reese and Miller (2006).

26.3 Vitamin deficiency

Vitamin A deficiency: The deficiency symptoms are usually not observed in commercial and pasture based production system. In backyard and free range system, the deficiency of vitamin A is common in tropical countries. Symptom include anorexia, poor growth rate, incoordination, trembling, spasms, paralysis, eye lesions and poor night vision. In breeder sow, farrow of blind, eyeless, weak, or malformed pigs are commonly seen.

Vitamin D deficiency: The sign includes rickets, osteomalacia, lameness, stiffness, weak and bent bones, fracture of long bones and posterior paralysis.it occurs due to insufficient calcium in the diet or a calcium/phosphorus imbalance. It is also seen in pigs reared in intensive system due to limited access to the sun, which reduces natural vitamin D production.

Vitamin E/Selenium deficiency: Also called Mulberry heart disease. Vitamin E and selenium are closely related as both protect cells from the detrimental effects of oxidation. Vitamin E prevents the formation of harmful free radicals while selenium destroy peroxides, another harmful compound. Selenium in this way prevent some deficiency symptoms of vitamin E. Both nutrients are required by the body and their deficiency symptoms are similar. Deficiency symptoms are anorexia, depression with muscle dystrophy and weakness, lowered body temperature poor reproduction and impaired immune system. Icterus, difficult locomotion, peripheral cyanosis, dyspnoea, weak pulse, hepatic necrosis, degenerative myopathy, oedema, yellow discoloration of adipose tissue. May cause sudden death in recently weaned piglets.

Vitamin K deficiency: Deficiency increases blood clotting time and pig may die due to haemorrhages. Certain components in mouldy feed and excessive levels of dietary calcium interfere with vitamin K activity, causing these signs.

Thiamine deficiency: Deficiency symptom include reduced appetite and body weight, vomiting, weak pulse, subnormal body temperature, nervous signs, sudden death due to heart failure.

Riboflavin deficiency: Deficiency symptom include anoestrous in post pubertal gilt. Sows exhibit anorexia and farrow pre mature dead pigs. Growing pigs show anorexia, poor growth and feed efficiency, rough hair coat, dermatitis, alopecia, stiffness, unsteady gait, scours, ulcerative colitis, inflammation of anal mucosa, vomiting, cataracts, light sensitivity and decreased immune response.

Niacin deficiency: Deficiency symptom include diarrhoea, weight loss, loss of appetite, weakness, rough skin and coat, dermatitis on the ears, exfoliate type dermatitis, hair loss, degeneration of nervous system.

Pantothenic acid deficiency: Deficiency symptom include goose-stepping gait, ataxia, anorexia and a non-infectious bloody diarrhoea. Necrotic enteritis, ulceration and haemorrhages in the large intestine, Bloody faeces may also observed.

Pyridoxine deficiency: Deficiency symptom include anorexia, decreased growth, dermatitis, diarrhoea, rough hair coat, scaly skin.

Choline deficiency: Deficiency symptom include incoordination, abnormal shoulder conformation, poor conformation (short legs, pot-belly), reduced litter size and may give birth to splay legged pigs.

Biotin deficiency: Deficiency symptom include excessive hair loss, dry and rough dermatitis with brown exudate, skin ulcerations and dermatitis, exudates around the eyes, inflammation of the mucous membranes of the mouth, transverse cracking of the hooves, and cracking or bleeding of the footpads.

Vitamin B12 deficiency: Deficiency symptom appeared in neonatal pigs fed synthetic diets low in vitamin B12 show hyperirritability, voice failure, pain and incoordination in the hindquarters.

Table 26.2: Deficiency symptoms of vitamins in swine.

Nutrients	*Deficiency symptoms*
Vitamin A	Anorexia, poor growth rate, poor night vision, incoordination and infertility
Vitamin D	Lameness, rickets, osteomalacia, fractures and swollen joints
Vitamin E	Anorexia, depression, muscular weakness, poor reproduction impaired immune system, udder oedema and agalactia, dysentery, respiratory disease and sudden death
Vitamin K	Increases blood clotting time, pig may die due to haemorrhages
Thiamine (B1)	Reduced appetite and body weight, vomiting, weak pulse, subnormal body temperature, nervous signs and sudden death due to heart failure

Riboflavin (B2)	Anoestrous in post pubertal gilt, pre mature dead pigs, anorexia, poor growth and feed efficiency, alopecia and dermatitis, stiffness and unsteady gait, scours and decreased immune response.
Pantothenic acid (B5)	Goose-stepping gait, ataxia, non-infectious bloody diarrhoea necrotic enteritis, ulceration and haemorrhages in the large intestine
Pyridoxine (B6)	Anorexia, reduced growth, dermatitis, diarrhoea, rough hair coat and scaly skin.
Biotin	Excessive hair loss, dry and rough dermatitis with brown exudate, skin ulcerations and dermatitis, transverse cracking of the hooves and cracking or bleeding of the footpads.
Choline	Incoordination, abnormal shoulder conformation, poor conformation (short legs, pot-belly), reduced litter size and birth of splay legged pigs
Folic acid	Anaemia, small litter size and reduced growth
Nicotinamide (Niacin)	Diarrhoea, weight loss, loss of appetite, rough skin and coat dermatitis on the ears, degeneration of nervous system

26.4 Mineral deficiency

Minerals are essential component that influence the efficiency of production. It is essential for optimal growth and physiologic function in pigs. Thus, it is mandatory to provide minerals as dietary supplements to promote efficient and profitable swine production in tropics.Signs of mineral deficiency diseases are shown in table 26.3.

Iron and copper deficiency: Sow colostrum and milk contains very low iron. Also, piglets has little reserve of iron. Suckling piglet has rapid growth and increase of blood volume hence deficiency of iron and anaemia will develop unless another source of iron is made available. Small amount of copper is required for utilization of iron by the body. Copper deficiency has similar symptoms as iron i.e. anaemia.

Deficiency reduce the rate of haemoglobin formation and cause anaemia in suckling pigs. Low haemoglobin and RBC count, pale mucous membranes, skin oedema about the neck and shoulders, listlessness, and spastic breathing (thumps). At necropsy, enlargement of the heart and spleen, hydropericardium, ascites, oedema in various tissues and fatty changes in the liver are seen.

Calcium and phosphorus deficiency: Deficiency symptom include rickets in growing pigs and osteomalacia in mature pigs. Deformity and bending of long bones and lameness in young pigs, and fractures and posterior paralysis in older pigs. Signs are similar to deficiency of vitamin D.

Iodine deficiency: Deficiency symptom include goitre (enlarged thyroid glands) which may not be apparently visible but can be observed at necropsy. Birth of weak or dead pigs with devoid (or less) of hair, mucinous oedema especially over enlarged foreparts of the body and oedematous tongue usually protrude from mouth.

Zinc deficiency: Deficiency symptom include parakeratosis in growing pigs in which there is dermatitis behind and at the base of the ears, on the inner side of the legs and along the abdomen. Later, skin becomes thickened, forming pimple-like projections (appear like hog mange mite) from which serum ooze out and crust is formed. Unbalanced ration that has excessive calcium, excessive phytic acid (sometimes present in soybean protein) or a low concentration of essential fatty acids will lead to zinc deficiency.

Salt (NaCl) deficiency: Deficiency symptom include poor growth, decreased feed intake, poor hair and skin condition and attempting to consume urine of other pigs.

Table 26.3.Signs of mineral deficiency diseases

Elements	*Deficiency Disease*
Iron and copper	Anaemia, low haemoglobin and RBC count, pale mucous membranes, skin oedema about the neck and shoulders, listlessness, and spastic breathing (thumps). At necropsy, enlargement of the heart and spleen, hydropericardium, ascites, oedema in various tissues and fatty changes in the liver.
Calcium and phosphorus	Rickets, osteomalacia, deformity and bending of long bones and lameness in young pigs, and fractures and posterior paralysis in older pigs.
Iodine	Goitre, birth of weak or dead pigs with devoid (or less) of hair, mucinous oedema especially over enlarged foreparts of the body and oedematous tongue usually protrude from mouth.
Zinc	Parakeratosis.
Salt (NaCl)	Poor growth, decreased feed intake, poor hair and skin condition and attempting to consume urine of other pigs.

26.5 Toxicoses in Swine

Aflatoxicosis

Aflatoxins are mycotoxins which is produced by Aspergillus flavus, Aspergillus parasiticus or Penicillium puberulum. It is produced when grains like corn, peanuts and soybeans are stored in poor (high moisture and temperature) condition. Major toxins produced are B1, B2, G1 and G2 in which B1 is potent hepatotoxin. The occurrence is in many parts of world and it effects depends on many factors but age is very important. Young pigs are more susceptible. Toxin reduce protein synthesis that affects pig growth and weakens their immune system.

Symptoms: Depend on the dose, length of exposure, and age of the pigs. The symptoms include reduce feed intake, average daily gain and feed efficiency, haemorrhage, hairy pigs, jaundice, weak immune response and agalactia in lactating sows.

Ergotism: The toxicosis caused by three major alkaloids produced by fungus of grasses and cereal grains, especially rye, oats and wheat namely Claviceps purpurea. These alkaloids cause arteriolar vasoconstriction and endothelial cell injury that often leads to thrombosis.

Symptoms: The symptoms include reduce feed intake, depression, vasoconstriction which lead to poor blood supply and cause bluish skin and gangrene of extremities (necrosis of tail and ears).

Fumonisin toxicosis

The toxicosis caused by toxin fumonisins mainly produced in corn by Fusarium moniliforme. It cause interstitial lung oedema and may lead to death. No effective treatment is available. The major symptoms are weak and pale pigs with slow growth, pulmonary oedema, short breath (dyspnoea), cyanosis, productive coughing, reproductive failure and sudden death.

Trichothecene toxicosis

The toxicosis caused by toxic compounds produced by certain Fusarium species that are classified as trichothecene mycotoxins. These toxins are immunosuppressive. The major symptoms are refuse to take feed, salivation and vomiting. Chronic cases may show paresis and seizure.

❑❑❑

Chapter 27

Abnormalities in Swine

—Dr. Kiros Abebe & Dr. Muuz Gebru

27.1 Hernias

Inguinal and scrotal hernia: The inguinal hernias are developmental defects in swine and have low heritability. Inguinal hernia may be unilateral (mostly occurring in left side) or bilateral and are believed to inherited polygenically in males. Scrotal hernia are beloved to be inherited by at least two pairs of genes and its heritability of liability appears to be in excess of 0.5. This condition prevails due to weak musculature that surrounds the inguinal canal. There is invagination of intestinal loop or other abdominal organs into the inguinal canal (inguinal hernia) or extended into the scrotum (scrotal hernia).

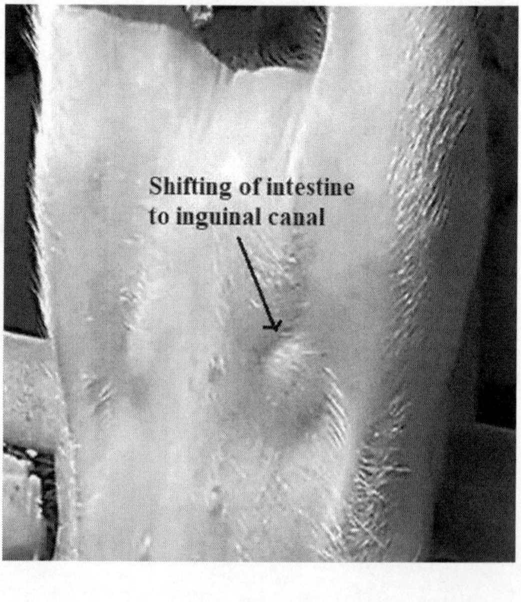

Figure 27.1: Inguinal hernia in pig.

The inguinal hernia are also commonly occurring during castration. In non-castrated males, generally pig remain unaffected but sometimes strangulation of the intestine within an inguinal hernia may occur.

Umbilical hernia: Also called belly bust or belly rupture. This condition may occur due to naval infection due to poor umbilical cord management at birth or naval suckling by pen mates.

Weaker musculature around naval area resulting in is invagination of intestinal loop or other abdominal organs into abdominal wall. Generally no adverse symptoms are observed but sometimes pig may die due to strangulation of the intestine. The genetic association of this condition is not well known but it is magnified by crowding to conserve heat during cold weather. Culling and surgical correction is not recommended.

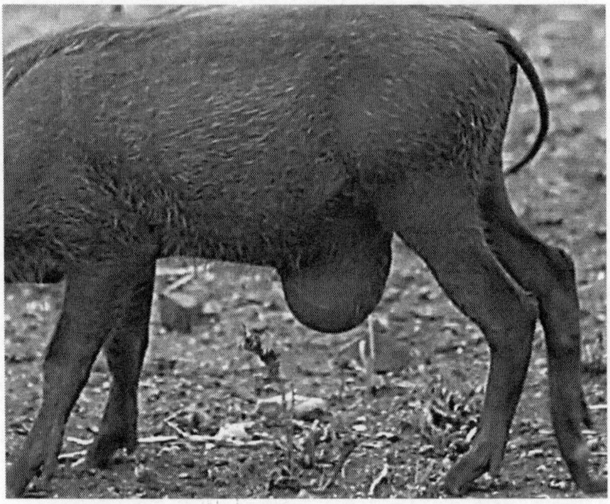

Figure 27.2: Umbilical hernia in pig.

27.2 Atresia ani

In this condition the pig is born without rectal opening. Female piglets may defecate through vulva (opening made from rectum to vagina) but male piglet usually die unless anal opening is made surgically. The actual cause is not known but believed to have a genetic cause hence culling of affected pigs and their parents are recommended. The abdomen of affected piglets increases in size and the die.

27.3 Cryptorchidism

When the male pig has one or no testicles in the scrotal sac (does not descent from abdominal cavity) is called cryptorchids or ridglings. When only one testis is descended (figure 27.3), they behave as normal. If both the testicles are not descended then the pig is sterile.

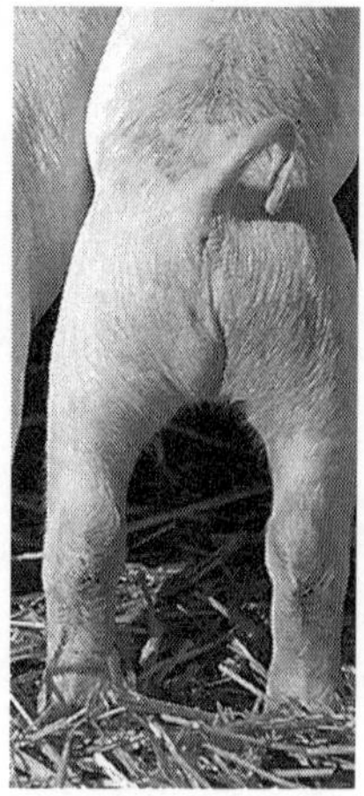

Figure 27.3: Cryptorchid pig with one testis in scrotal sac.

This condition is sex-limited and believed to be polygenic (at least two pairs of genes are responsible). Culling of affected pig and their parents recommended.

27.4 Hermaphrodites

Hermaphrodites are mostly female pig (XX genotype) which has altered chromosome due to translocation of portion of Y chromosome on X or mutation in the X chromosome that has removed the depressing effect of maleness that is thought to exist on the normal X chromosome. It is frequently seen in Large White and Landrace breeds of pig. Condition is genetic hence the affected pig and their parents are usually culled.

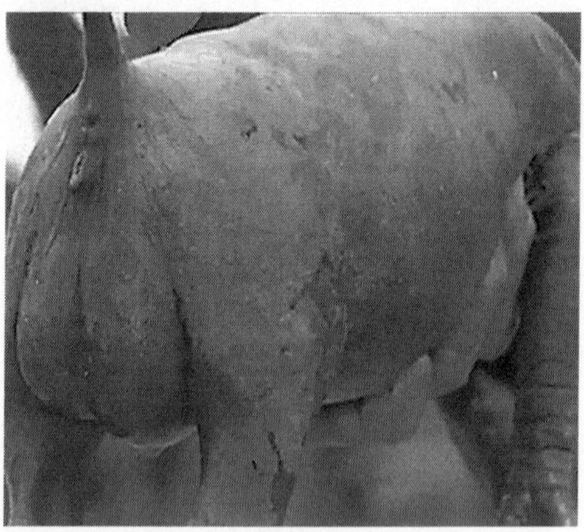

Figure 27.4: Hermaphrodite pig.

27.5 Nipple Abnormalities

Inverted nipples: In this condition, nipples are not protrude out from the udder surface. Inward teat canal is prevent the flow of milk and the teat is not utilized for suckling. This condition is believed to have genetic cause but the number of involved genes are not known.

Blind nipples: In this condition, there is no opening of teat canal. The aberration of teat with the rough floor surface is the main cause of this problem. As cause is non-genetic, culling is not recommended.

27.6 Tremors

Synonym: Myoclonia congenita, trembles, shivers, shakers, or jumpy pig disease

Tremors in pig are mostly present at birth but certain forms are often first expressed at later ages or few hours after birth. It is characterized by rhythmic twitching of the neck and legs. The piglets with minor symptoms are able to move and nurse. Piglets with severe tremors unable to move and die due to starvation, chilling, and crushed by the sow. One of the cause of tremors is porcine circovirus as it is isolated from the affected case but it is also considered to be under genetic control.

27.7 Neonatal Diarrhoea

It is caused by Escherichia coli bacteria that cause high morbidity and mortality in neonatal piglets. There is sudden onset and piglets has watery or pasty diarrhoea and they become dehydrated, lethargy and develops systemic infection. E. coli have cell-surface antigens and it attached to the glycoprotein receptors on the intestinal wall of piglets. After attachment, bacteria multiple and release enterotoxins which cause diarrhoea. Certain piglets lack the intestinal receptor for the K88 strain (single-locus autosomal recessive trait) of Escherichia coli and are resistant to K88 bacteria and to diarrhea caused by K88 strains.

❑❑❑

Chapter 28

Techniques of Necropsy Diagnoses in Swine

—Dr. Yohannes T. Asfaw

28.1 Overview of Swine Production

Largely due to the increase in worldwide demand for meat, pigs have become a crucial food source due to their fast growth, efficient feed conversion, quick turnover, and prolificacy (FAO, 2017). Pork is the most consumed meat from terrestrial animals, accounting for over 37 percent of global meat intake, followed closely by chicken (35.2%) and beef (21.6%) (FAO, 2013). Due to the increased demand, the pig sector has grown steadily over the past decades as indicated (Figure 1) though the distribution of pigs is largely influenced by religious and cultural factors (FAO, 2017). For instance, limited number of pigs are found in countries where Muslim and Orthodox Christian religions are dominantly practiced.

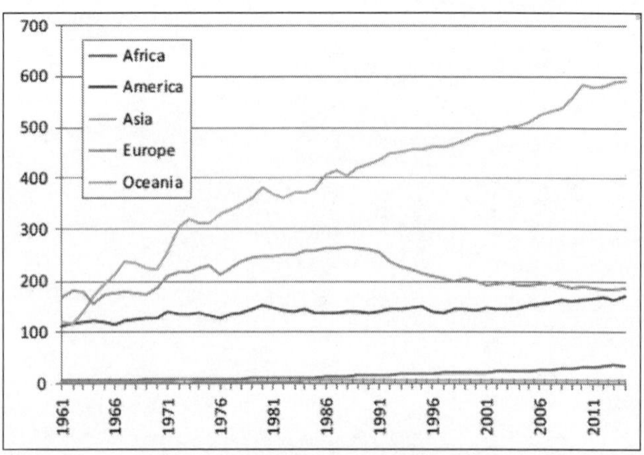

Figure 1: Number of pigs (x1 000 000) in the world by regions (1961-2014)
Source: FAOSTATA, 2016

The sector is characterized by a deep divide between traditional, small-scale, subsistence productions on the one hand, and industrialized pig farming with increasing vertical integration on the other. Of course, there is a whole range of intermediate systems in between. Commercial pig production has intensified significantly in recent decades. More pigs of the same few breeds are kept on fewer, larger farms, with corresponding increased output of animal products. Large-scale production systems have achieved a high level of uniformity because they are based on the same genetic material and therefore use similar feed and housing infrastructure. But while these larger-scale operations are helping meet an increasing share of global pork demand, about 43 percent of pigs are still produced in backyard and other small-scale settings, particularly in the developing world (Robinson et al., 2011). In the developing world, most pigs are still kept in traditional, small-scale, subsistence production systems in which they provide much more than meat. In such low-input systems, pigs produce added value for farmers by converting household waste into protein, while also providing manure to fertilize fields and fishponds. Hence, pork contributes to food security and nutrition, while live animals represent a financial safety net, play a significant role in cultural traditions, and supply additional cash for school fees, medical treatment, and small investments.

In both production systems, the level of priorities in adjusting production practices or investing in biosecurity to prevent and control pig diseases could vary. Indeed, the backyard sector, characterized by low biosecurity, outdated husbandry practices and technologies, and poor awareness of, and compliance with, animal health regulations (outbreak reporting, movement control, certifications, vaccination, etc.) plays a major role in the introduction, spread, and maintenance of several pig diseases. However, in either of the two production systems, pig diseases are major problems of the sector significantly impacting the productivity and productivity of swine farms (FAO, 2017).

To tackle the impacts of swine diseases at the field level, early and proper diagnosis of cases is very critical tool that determines the success of treatment outcomes, also contribute for reducing unnecessary treatment costs and loss of animals. Moreover, animal health data obtained from necropsy are valuable information for national surveillance systems (species, breed, sex, weight, date, animal age (in days), how the animal died (e.g., euthanized) and address of the owner. Information about the clinical history of necropsied animals was not available in 99% of the reports and for this reason clinical history was excluded from study (Paul, 2008). Among swine disease diagnosis methods, it is necropsy that warranty the early and proper diagnosis of mortalities and morbidities of animals at farm levels. However, necropsy is area of expertise where knowledge and skill of pathology is required, and hence, performing necropsy is difficult job for many of veterinarians working at different fields. Therefore, this chapter aimed to help educate veterinary students, veterinarians and researchers to equip themselves with the techniques and tactics of performing necropsy based diagnosis of swine diseases during outbreaks and mortalities.

28.2 Necropsy Siagnosis in Swine

28.2.1 Definition of necropsy and its importance and usefulness

Necropsy is a Latin word which is to mean "Death examination" and it is a branch of pathology which studies gross pathologic lesions and all sort of abnormalities on died body. Hence, it is the recognition, description and interpretation of pathologic lesions or abnormalities at the clinical level of the whole died animal. It provides a rapid determination of potential problems which could correlate with clinical disease and support a presumptive diagnosis in light of the accompanying history and serve as a spring board for additional investigations if needed. This is because the gross lesions of some diseases are sufficiently distinct in their pattern to be presumptively diagnostic based upon necropsy alone and for many disorders, the gross morbid anatomy is highly suggestive of a particular disease or class of related diseases, and often the pattern of lesions suggests a pathogenesis or mechanisms of the clinical disease. However, the gross lesions are not distinct or specific and require additional diagnostic modalities to confirm or establish a diagnosis definitively. In this regard, necropsy is aroad mapfor what portions of the animal should be selected for histopathology, bacterial and fungal culture, virus isolation or toxin identification. Additionally, it provides a permanent, written and legal record of the medical problems of the patient.

For the above reasons, necropsy is very important and useful tool in veterinary practice in general and swine health in particular as it gives the following opportunities for pathologists, partitioning veterinarians, swine owners, researchers and other relevant actors in swine industry or value chain.

- Rapid determination of potential problems which often sufficiently distinct for presumptive diagnosis of a pathologic process such as inflammatory and neoplastic processes.
- It is also occasionally highly suggestive of specific disease with a pathognomic lesions.
- The lesion pattern may suggest mechanisms and pathogenesis a pathological condition
- Helps establishing facts in comparative pathology as related agents may cause similar lesions.
- It also guides or serve as "Road map" for what to culture or examine further. This helps as practical guideline for practitioners in making decisions on sample collection and selection of laboratory test.
- Good necropsy reports provide a permanent, legal record of the anatomic lesions in the patient and should correlate with the histopathologic, microbiological and toxicologic findings.

28.3 Current practices and limitations of Necropsy

Generally speaking, performance of the autopsy in veterinary medicine is unique in its execution when compared to human medicine where most of public and private veterinary practitioners do the necropsy themselves. Thus, it is important to understand the fundamentals of the necropsy to get the most out of it. The necropsy is an ephemeral event and when it's over, it's over!This makes the accurate description and interpretation of the necropsy findings critical because that is what remains in the permanent record as the basis for later historical, medical and legal review and interpretation. A principal limitation of retrospective clinical studies is a lack of or poorly conducted necropsy with inconsistent or incomplete characterization of the lesions (Paul, 2008).

Contrary to popular belief, the definitive diagnosis of disease is not always made at the microscopic level. The microscopic examination evaluates a tiny fraction of the organs and tissues. These histopathologic findings are integrated with the results of the autopsy and interpreted in light of the signalment, history, clinical appearance and laboratory tests to arrive at a diagnosis. What every histopathologist wants to know above all else is what the gross appearance was? This is easy when the pathologist performs both the autopsy and histopathologic examinations. However, the culture of veterinary medicine is such that most of the time the necropsy is performed by a clinician and the tissues are sent to a pathologist (often far away) for histopathology. To acquire precision and efficiency in the pathologic diagnosis of disease and maximize the results of the necropsy, the clinician must accurately observe, describe, record, interpret and communicate the results of the autopsy to the pathologist. When this is done properly, pathologists can maximize their contribution to the process often by providing not just a summary of the lesions they observe (called as morphologic diagnosis) but making a specific disease diagnosis. All too often veterinary students do not understand this. Although trained to perform the necropsy, clinicians do not assign sufficient importance to it or perform it often enough to reduce it to reliable practice and get the most out of it when needed. The things the pathologist most wants to know, indeed frequently needs to know, for definitive interpretation, are often out of his/her control. As a result communication between clinician and pathologist breaks down leaving all parties dissatisfied, including the swine owners who depend upon correct diagnosis for prognosis, decision making, grief counseling, absolution of guilt and closure. Clinicians are frustrated because they are getting only morphologic diagnoses which they cannot relate to clinical diseases instead of definitive clinical disease diagnoses which they understand and know how to treat or explain to their clients. Pathologists become frustrated because they know they can provide more but lack the information essential to make a definitive diagnosis (King et al., 2014; Paul, 2008).

28.4 Necropsy Procedures in Swine

Necropsy can be performed in many ways and the key to a successful necropsy is thoroughness and it must be ensured that all organs are examined and the important lesions discovered. However, availability of necessary necropsy equipment, skilled person (pathologist), standard necropsy procedures guarantee the outcome of every necropsy (King et al., 2014; Paul, 2008). Hence, before commencing the necropsy, the following equipment are required and hence, they must be made ready. It is very difficult to make necropsy unless the pathologist or anyone who is performing the necropsy is well equipped with the required equipment and materials.

- Standard post-mortem kit including boning and skinning knives, scissors, scalpel blades, forceps
- Large shears or pruning secateurs to cut through ribs and jaw, bone saw
- Shears or small axe and hammer for brain removal
- Dry swabs, swabs in media (viral transport media, Amies media/charcoal), specimen jars for individual fresh samples, 10% formalin, large containers for pooled formalin fixed samples
- Personal protection equipment – overalls, gloves, mask, eye protection
- Laboratory submission forms, permanent markers.

After ensuring availability of necessary materials, manpower, necropsy room or site, the swine necropsy will be proceed with the following stepwise procedures.

Here it must be noted that swine cadaver or live animal which is going to be necropsied should be officially and legally submitted to the necropsy facility by a farm owner or any legal representative of an institute in written request detailing the following information. Animal's ID, Species, Breed, Sex, and Age, Died/Killed/Unknown, Method of Euthanasia, Date and Time of Death, Total Number Affected, Duration of Illness, Clinical history: Describe clinical examination findings, Antemortem Diagnosis, Body Weight, name and address of Veterinarian in charge, name and address of Client, including the owner's signature for legal permission to do the necropsy. With this, three euthanized pigs with typical signs, acutely affected and untreated (if available) OR 3 freshly dead pigs will be necropsied. It is to bear in mind that selection of pigs for necropsy is the most important step in obtaining an accurate and timely diagnosis. While selecting pigs care must be taken that pigs that have been treated for days or weeks with antibiotics will be unrewarding if the goal of necrosis is to isolate pathogenic bacteria. Likewise, selecting only pigs that are chronically ill will skew the diagnostic picture, resulting in isolation only of common secondary or opportunistic pathogens and finding histopathological lesions masked by scarring or regeneration rather than the inciting lesion (Gramer et al., 2005). This is because selecting carefully to include acutely affected pigs will be the greatest help to the producer, the pathologist, and the veterinarian seeking treatment or prevention strategies.

If dead body is to be submitted, for best results, dead animals should be necropsied as soon as possible after death. If feasible, refrigerate animals until necropsy. This is because post-mortem changes begin immediately, hence, they create difficult in appropriately identify the ante mortem lesions. If the whole animal (dead or sick) cannot be submitted, collect and preserve specimens from the field for histopathological examination.

(A) External examination of the cadaver

Perform a thorough external examination of the skin, hooves, eyes, ears, nostrils, mouth and external genitalia. Palpate the joints and legs.

Write down any lesions or changes while keeping the following questions in mind (King et al., 2014; Paul, 2008; Gramer et al., 2005). Is the hair coat rough or shiny? Are there any skin lesions (redness, swelling, crusts, pustules, etc.)? Is there nasal or ocular discharge? Are there ulcers in the mouth, on the gingiva or tongue? Are the dorsal spinal processes showing or is the animal fat and in good flesh? Is the perineum stained with blood or diarrhea? Are the joints swollen? Is there swelling and redness of the coronary band above the hooves? Are the hooves cracked, worn, or smooth?

Sample skin lesions by collecting pieces of affected skin into a sterile container and into formalin. Swab discharges or collect a fresh sample of the exudate/fluid. Eyes and ears can be submitted whole in formalin for histopathology if they are abnormal. In cases of lameness or joint swelling, open and sample the affected joints and a selection of major joints (i.e. hip joints, carpal joints, tarsus, stifle, and elbow). Incise through the skin with a knife. Incise the joint capsule with a sterile scalpel and collect a sterile swab of joint fluid into Amies. Consider submitting the joint whole or a sample of joint capsule in formalin.

(B) Opening the cadaver

The cadaver need to be open and every organ will be removed and examined as follows (King et al., 2014; Paul, 2008; Gramer et al., 2005).

Position the pig right side down and Make a stab incision with the tip of the knife into the right axilla. Extend the skin excision cranially, cutting through the subcutaneous tissue and dermis so as not to dull the knife, just to the right of midline, to the chin, and caudally to the perineum, dorsal to the genitalia.

(i) Reflect back completely the right front and rear legs by cutting the muscles and tendons, disarticulating the hip joint and severing the muscular attachments of the scapula. Examine the musculature and hip joint. Sample hind limb skeletal muscle into formalin. Samples submitted in formalin should be <1cm thick.

(ii) Expose the abdominal cavity by carefully cutting the fascia and muscles along the last rib and along the back, then reflecting the tissue back. Pull up on the abdominal wall when cutting to avoid entering the stomach or intestines. The superficial inguinal lymph nodes will be revealed and can be examined for size and color. Then, the abdomen will be opened and reflect towards you; take care not to puncture the intestines.

(iii) Remove the ribs by cutting through the costalchondral junctions near the sternum. Dissect 2 or 3 ribs at a time and break them dorsally towards the vertebra to remove them. Note how difficult or easy it was to break the ribs as a general test of bone strength. Trim away the diaphragm and muscle to expose the thoracic cavity, lungs and heart.

(iv) Examine the visceral organs in the abdominal and thorax cavities in-situ. Record any abnormalities by writing a description and taking photographs. Look for peritoneal, pleural or pericardial exudate and if present collect any exudate into a sterile container or swab into Amies media.

(v) Skin underneath the neck and chin. Use shears to cut through the mandibular symphysis and split the lower jaw. Roll the head dorsally, split the lower jaw apart. Grasp and pull the tongue backwards while cutting the soft tissues along both mandibles.

(vi) Examine the oral cavity. If there are oral lesions present such as vesicles, ulcers collect a sample into formalin, swabs into Amies, and swabs or epithelial tags into viral transport media or into a sterile container. Vesicular fluid can be aspirated and placed in a plain blood tube. Sample the tonsils. The tonsils are the pitted, textured area of the soft palate outlined below. Using scissors, remove the tonsils. Place half into formalin and half into a sterile container. Grasp the tongue and pull it caudally.

(vii) Cut the hyoid bones, dissect along the trachea and oesophagus into the chest and remove the thoracic viscera all together. You will need to cut through the oesophagus, aorta and caudal vena cava where they pass through the diaphragm. Examine the trachea, oesophagus, bronchial lymph nodes, lungs, pericardium and heart. Open the trachea and main stem bronchi. Bread slice the lungs to ensure lesions deep in the lung are not missed. Collect thin sections (no greater than 1cm thick) of lung, trachea, bronchial lymph node, oesophagus and any lesions into formalin. Collect a 3cm cube of fresh lung into a sterile container. If bronchial lymph nodes are enlarged or obvious, collect a fresh sample into a sterile container.

(viii) Examine the pericardium and heart upon cutting through the ventricles. Collect a 'T-shaped' section of heart which includes left and right ventricular free wall and interventricular septum and add this to the formalin pot. The tissue should be <1cm thick. Open the left and right ventricles and incise up into the atria and great vessels. Examine the heart valves. Sample any lesions into a sterile jar and into formalin and swab any exudates into Amies.

(ix) Examine the tracheobronchial lymph nodes, sternal lymph nodes, and submandibular lymph nodes. Note if they are enlarged or hemorrhagic. Collect lymph nodes for cultures and slice some thinly for histopathology.

(x) In the abdomen, examine the spleen. Collect a 3cm cube of spleen into a sterile container and a thin section (<1cm) into formalin.

(xi) Cut the diaphragm away from the body wall. Grasp the mesenteric root and pull the viscera caudally, lifting the intestines and liver out of the abdomen and cutting the mesentery. The kidneys and urogenital tract should remain in the abdomen. Leaving the colon as the last point of attachment, incise the colon as far caudally as possible and collect a faecal sample.

(xii) Dissect the liver from the intestines. Examine and bread slice the organ. Collect a 3x3cm fresh sample of liver into a sterile container and a <1cm thick section into formalin.

(xiii) Spread out the intestine by cutting through the mesenteric root. Identify and examine the ileum, caecum and ileocaecal junction for presence of any lesions. Collect a 5cm long section of ileum and place half into formalin and half into a sterile container. Collect an ileocaecal lymph node into both formalin and a sterile container. Examine the remaining sections of the intestinal tract. Examine the small and large intestine. Open sections of all areas of the intestinal tract and examine the mucosa, especially in cases of diarrhoea. If there are abnormal contents or areas of mucosa target these areas; collect fresh intestinal contents or swabs in Amies. Collect short segments of duodenum, jejunum, caecum and colon. Take care not to scrape the mucosal surface of pieces of tissue placed into formalin

(xiv) Open the stomach and examine the mucosa. Collect a sample of stomach contents into a sterile container and a piece of stomach into formalin.

(xv) Remove both kidneys, cut in half length ways and examine the cortex, medulla and pelvis. Collect a 3x3cm piece of kidney into a sterile container. Collect a thin piece of kidney which includes cortex, medulla and pelvis into formalin.Examine the bladder. If there is evidence of urogenital disease, collect a sample of bladder into formalin and a urine sample into a sterile container.

(xvi) Examine the urogenital tract i.e. ovaries and uterus or testes and check presence of pathologic lesions. Bread slice these tissues. Collect fresh and fixed samples if required.

(xvii) Remove the brain. Saw or split the head sagittally in a large pig or remove the calavarium with shears in a small pig. Collect a sample of fresh brain into a sterile container. A small piece of cortex (olfactory lobe or occipital cortex) is sufficient. Alternatively, collect a meningeal swab. The rest of the brain should be submitted whole in formalin.If there is a history of neurological signs, consider collecting additional samples such as spinal cord and peripheral nerve.

Finally after thoroughly examining each and every organ in situ and ex situ, the cadaver must be properly disposed so as to not be source of infection for future and abate the risk of environmental contamination. Indicate preferred method for disposing of remains.

(xviii) Moreover, all of the collected samples should be labelled clearly and they should be submitted appropriately with a completed submission form to respective laboratory. The best specimen for submission is a recently euthanized untreated animal that exhibited typical clinical signs.

(C) Necropsy Report

Record the necropsy findings along with the reported clinical signs, diagnosis along with list of differential diagnoses or concerns. Be sure to include a history of vaccinations and treatments if they are known. To proceed with reporting of the necropsy findings back to the client, skill and experiences determines the ability of a pathology or other expert to recognize significant lesions and obtain a diagnosis. Hence, it is of great interest to study and internalize how the descriptions and interpretations of gross lesions visualized, palpated and found on incisions during necropsy are made.

28.5 Descriptions and Interpretations of Gross lesions during Necropsy

Complete description or recording of what someone observed is the one of central goals of necropsy. However, everything about the interpretation of the described lesions is entirely dependent upon the experience and skill of the expert who performs the necropsy (King et al., 2013). In this regards, the art of necropsy diagnosis is of two critical sequential process, i.e. description and interpretations. Gross observations (descriptions) of lesions are objective and never change while interpretations are subjective, open to discussion and can be altered. This shows that interpretation is always a guess of a pathologistbut it can be a very good guess depending on the level of experiences and skills of that pathologist. However, it highly advisable to "Always justify your interpretation by accurate descriptions"!

Example, one can have the following description and interpretations of given lesions of lung recording during necropsy.

Lesion description	*Lesion interpretation*
The lung was diffuse dark red to plum colored, heavy, wet and foamy fluid freely ran from the cut surface. It felt firmer than normal and not Crepitate	Diffuse pulmonary congestion and edema Diffuse acute interstitial pneumonia

28.5.1 Fundamental Elements of Lesion description during Necropsy

The description of gross lesions begins with the observation and characterization of the abnormal findings. To do this one must know what attributes are important and what they mean when observed. The following is a list of those attributes which are elements of a good gross descriptions of abnormalities seen at necropsy (King et al., 2014; Paul, 2008; Gramer et al., 2005).

- Distribution – A spatial arrangement pattern. What is the spatial arrangement of lesions?
- Demarcation – Distinct or indistinct. How clearly set off from the adjacent is it?
- Contour – Raised, flat, or depressed. Are the lesions raised, flat or depressed?
- Shape –Do the lesions have a geometric shape?
- Color - "Well, what color is it?"
- Size – Absolute vs relative. absolute vs. relative; lesion, whole organ, paired organs
- Texture – Cut surface; amorphous or solid. What does the cut surface look like? Amorphous or solid
- Consistency – Fluid, soft, firm, hard, gritty. How does the lesion feel?
- Special Features – odor, sound
- Extent - % of the organ affected. How much of the organ or tissue is affected?
- Chronicity- A subjective assessment; usually difficult to be precise.

For easily memorizing, please see, the following methodological descriptions and interpretations of lesions.

<u>Morphological descriptions and interpretations of lesions may include the following:</u>

Distribution:	Organ(s) Unilateral – Bilateral Focal – Multifocal (Disseminated) Locally Extensive – Diffuse Whole Body – Localized Generalized
Time:	Peracute – Acute – Subacute – Chronic – Chronic Active
Severity:	Minimal Moderate Marked Slight Severe
Cause:	Verminous – Bacterial – Chemical – Viral – Traumatic – Protozoal – Mycotic – Toxic – etc.
Type:	Croupous – Hemorrhagic – Purulent – Fibrinous – Fibrinopurulent – etc.

A. Distribution

The spatial arrangement of the lesions in the organ or tissue is important because distribution may reflect pathogenesis. Lesions or abnormalities may occur with distinct distribution patterns which when recognized are clues to the disease process and assist in estimating severity or significance of the observed findings. Among the attributes of gross lesions, distribution is one of the most important which should be included in every morphologic diagnosis. For instance, in many dermatopathies, the lesion distribution is the key to diagnosis. The distribution of the gross lesions could be of random, symmetrical, focal, multi focal, multifocal coalescing, military, diffuse and segmental type. And this type of distribution of lesions is helpful in interpreting the lesions.

Random distribution of lesions: This happens when the lesion occurs without reference to architectureor relationship to particular organ or tissue structures. The scattering of abscesses or tumors throughout a lung or liver may be random. Hence, a distribution seemingly determined by chance. As part of the random distribution, there is haphazard random distribution of lesions which is non-consistently associated with certain structures in the organ or tissue, easy to see, not specific with respect to cause or pathogenesis. Many pathologic processes often appear to occur randomly this way.

Symmetrical distribution of lesions: This is a pattern with some degree of organization or architectural form is apparent in the abnormality. May have a geometric shape which sis non-random and bilateral symmetry. Occurs when a pathologic process highlights an anatomic or physiologic subunit of the organ or tissue. Often defined by vascular beds, lobules, ducts, airways, tubules. Bilateral lesions may imply a metabolic disorder affecting a certain group of related cells present in distinctly separated areas of the organ or tissue or the same location in paired organs. Asymmetrical or organized appearance occurs when a pathologic process highlights or outlines a certain anatomic or physiologic subunit; often it outlines a vascular unit or circulatory bed. Airways in the lung, portal tracts in the liver, glomeruli or tubules in kidney. Bilateral lesions may with similar physiological sensitivity to a metabolic disorder of redundant tissue on both sides of the midline

Focal distribution of lesion: It is a single defined lesion on a backgroundwhich is either normal or itself abnormal but containing or reflecting a different process than present in the focal lesion. I.e. a solitary tumor in the liver; an abscess in a congested lung. One of the easiest distributions to see but with little discriminative power as to pathogenesis.

Multifocal distribution of lesions: This is defined as more than a single discrete lesions are produced on a background of the organ or tissue. It is widely and highly variable with several to many lesions and having abnormality in 2 or 3 or more foci. Such multi focal distribution of lesions suggests an embolic shower which is also easy to appreciate. Under this category, there is Multifocal to Coalescing distribution of lesions when there are many lesions present that may appear to be growing together or fusing. This reflects an active process which is expanding or not otherwise contained or limited by the host defense mechanisms. Several to many focal lesions that appear to be growing together or fusing. Additionally, there is a Miliary type of distribution of lesions which is a special case of multifocaldistribution of lesionsin which there are numerous tiny foci present that are too numerous to count. The miliary pattern stems from amiliariuswhich is a Latin word for millet seed. Miliary distributions may reflect a recent embolic shower to the organ or tissue. Because the lesions are small, the implication is that the event is recent.

Segmental distribution of lesions: It is a well-defined portion or segment of the tissue is abnormal; sometimes with a distinct geometric shape. This distribution implies that the pathologic process is restricted by anatomic or physiologic factors and so occupies a discrete portion. Such segmental lesions often define a vascular bed.

Diffuse distribution of lesions: This show that everythingin the frame of reference is abnormal or affected.This generally implies that is with greater severity and therefore having higher significance than focal or multifocal lesions. Also because it takes time for a process to affect the entire tissue, diffuse lesions may (but not necessarily) be more chronic or older. And it is often difficult to appreciate because there is no contrast with normal.

B. Demarcation of lesions

It show the degree to which the lesion is set off or defined from the adjacent tissue. With this definition, the lesions reported during necropsy could be well demarcated or poorly demarcated, as described below.

Well demarcated: The boundary between normal and abnormal is abrupt, discrete and easily seen.This implies that the lesion represents a different tissue or is well contained or separated from the adjacent normal tissue. Tumors, abscesses with capsules, pus, a rim of necrosis often produce a well demarcated lesion.

Poorly Demarcated: The boundary between normal and abnormal is blurred or not easily seen. This implies that the lesion and adjacent tissue may be similar; the process gradually infiltrates into normal or may be poorly contained.

C. Contour

Contour is the degree to which the lesion is elevated or depressed with respect to the adjacent tissue. It can be of raised, depressed or flat lesions produced on a ground of an organ or tissue. Raised implies that something is addedto the organ or tissue to cause expansion. For instance, it could happen in cases of fluids such as blood, transudates, exudates, effusions, edema, urine accumulation, gas in the form of emphysema, cells which could be. Hyperplasia, abnormal (neoplasia), exudates (inflammation), stroma such as fibrous tissue, cartilage, bone or foreign material (i.e. plant material, parasites). Similarly, depressed contour implies that something is removed or lost.Most commonly this is related to necrosis or atrophy but remember some organs are physiologically dynamic like lung, spleen, urinary bladder. The most common thing taken away from the lung is air. On the other hand, Flat contour is when the lesion is neither raised nor depressed with respect to the surrounding tissues. This may imply either a recent event which has not had sufficient time to progress or a process that does not cause expansion or necrosis.

D. Shape

Shape describes the geometric figure of the lesion's resemblance and hence, the shape of lesion will be judged as circular, rectangular, triangular, spherical etc. Because the vasculature of tissues is often laid out in geometric patterns or distinct shapes may reflect a pathologic process highlighting or outlining a vascular bed such as infarcts or segmental lesions. Moreover, symmetrical shapes or patterns which appear somewhat organized rather than random may reflect a unit of architecture such as lobes, lobules, septae, hepatic portal tracts.

E. Color

Color is one of the most obvious attributes of a lesion, especially when the lesion differs from the normal color. Normal color of a tissue or organ is determined by the innate color or number of cells and stroma in that tissue. Often this is colorless or white, special pigments or adipose tissue i.e. myelin, myoglobin, steroids, bile, and the amount of blood present in the vascular bed your eye sees the net effect of these 3 characteristics. For instance, dark tissues such as muscle, spleen and liver have high pigment/tissue ratio. Light Tissues such as lung and brain have low pigment/tissue ratio or high fat content. Red to Reddish Black usually means blood or hemoglobin pigment indicate that the tissue is in congestion or hemorrhage state. Congestion tends to be a wider spread phenomenon than hemorrhage and tends to be poorly demarcated. White to Gray or Yellow color often the lack of blood and hence, indicates necrosis is often pale because of the lack of blood. Moreover, exudates are also white to yellow and because Exudates add something, foci of exudation are often raised. Additionally, fibrosis is pale to white but because scar tissue fills in areas of necrosis (something removed) and contracts as it matures, foci of fibrosis are often depressed. Similarly, hyperplasia and Neoplasia often light to white or the normal tissue color; granulation tissue is pink early when it has abundant capillaries; white as it matures. Bilirubin stained tissues (icterus) may be yellow *Yellow discoloration in the CNS may indicate malacia

Green color often bile or bile pigments and it can be seen as post mortem bile staining of tissue.

Termed as Pseudo-melanosis: Coagulation necrosis may be various shades of green, Eosinophilic inflammation may impart a greenish discoloration to tissues, Aspiration pneumonia with plant material Pigmented fungi can give a green color. On top of that, Pseudo-melanosis (Artificial staining of tissues post mortem by bile from the gall bladder and H2S pigments from the gastrointestinal tract, usually limited penetration into organ adjacent to liver or bowel stain green black. Interestingly, pathological conditions such as aspiration pneumonia (due to the action of saprophytic bacteria) is seen with green black discoloration.

Black –Brown: Black usually means melanin where Melanosis is flat, not enough to create contour while Melanoma is raised where proliferating cells create contour. The tissue or organ may look brown due to presence of pigmented fungisuch as Cladosporium and Curvularia produce which produce brown color i.e. hemosiderin.

"The Fine Arts 101 Rule of Colors" i.e."Processes producing a dark color (congestion, hemorrhage) can mask processes producing a light color (necrosis, inflammation)"

F. Size

A size matters in describing gross lesions as it explains how big is the lesion or abnormal area. Hence, measuring or otherwise estimate the size of lesions as this directly impacts the significance. While doing this, the sizes of dimensions of masses, nodules, flat foci, depressions need to be measured or estimated. The size implies that small lesions are more recent events than large ones and may be less important. In case of multiple lesions, they may be of uniform or non-uniform size. Uniform size lesions are lesions of the same size while non-uniform size are lesions are of differing size. This uniform seizes of lesions may mean the pathologic events have occurred over a short period or at the same time and are progressing at the same rate. On the other hand the non-uniform size lesions may mean the pathologic events are separated in time or have different rates of progression, i.e. the small lesions are more recent, the larger lesions are older; recurring pathologic process such as multiple waves of metastasis.

The size of lesion could be discrete of whole organ. Unlike discrete lesions, organ size is often relative and difficult to seebecause of the lack of contrast; often a subjective opinion. Easiest to appreciate with paired organs but small differences in organ size may not be perceptible, i.e. hearts, livers, adrenal glands. Hence, "The Organ Size Rule" i.e. "Always give more weight to objective evaluations than to subjective evaluations". The organ size could be larger than normal because something is added in case of hyperplasia, edema, neoplasia, congestion, inflammation. On the other hand, smaller than normal is when something is removed/lostmay be due to hypoplasia, atrophy, and necrosis. In case of paired organs or tissues, it matters when there is difference in sizes where one of the affected organ is larger or small size than the other. While dealing of size of organs or tissue, additional attributes such as shape, color, symmetry and contour are fundamentally important in describing and properly interpreting the lesions.

It is also very important to learn the dynamism of the size of some organs which are physiologically dynamic i.e. they change size and shape for functional reasons or in response to physiologic demands. Hence, lungs, urinary bladder Air and urine within the organs are rapidly dynamic.

G. Texture

Texture describes the appearances of the cut surface in an organ or tissue look like. Hence, the texture of the lesion could be amorphous or solid. Amorphous type of texture is a semisolid, unorganized, no architecture, cannot hold shape and not cohesive. It is something when someone spread it with a butter knifeand this type of texture describe pathological conditions such as pus, exudates and liquefactive necrosis. On the other hand, solid texture lesions organs or tissues have apparent structure or architecture, holds together or maintains shape, not spreadable with a butter knife unlike the lesions having amorphous textureandthey are usually means viable, living cells and tissue or stroma. Hyperplasia, neoplasia, stromal deposition.

"The Texture Caveat", i.e. "Sometimes granulomatous inflammation looks like neoplasia" (Non-caveating granulomatous inflammation may be "cohesive")

H. Consistency

Consistency of a lesion describes how that lesion fees when it is palpated by hand. Accordingly, the consistency of a lesion could be gaseous/air trapped in tissue (e.g. Emphysema), fluid in tissue and feels wet or squishy/ like a water balloon and this means edema, blood, transudates, fluid rich exudates, effusions, urine. The consistency could also be soft when the tissue is fluid rich/cell or stroma poor indicating exudates, firm when the tissue is fluid poor/cell or stroma rich reflecting exudates, hyperplasia, neoplasia, scar tissue or fibrosis, and hard usually means mineralized stroma or matrix; cartilage, bone, calcified tissues. To better describe the consistency of a lesion, it is advised to learn that fluids (serous, water, urine, transudates edema) takes the shape of its container and you can pour it, while serosanguinous is clear but blood tinged and it is a common postmortem finding in body cavities. On the other hand, sero-fibrinous to fibrinous is a cloudy with strands of opaque white to yellow, and chylous is a milky white indicating lymph. Finally, a purulentto sero-purulent lesion is an opaque, thin to thick and contains degenerate neutrophils e.g. pus.

I. Special Features

Special features such as weight, sound and odor of a lesion are also important attributes in lesion description. The relative and subjective weight of an organ or a tissue though it is often subtle and difficult to objectively may determine whether the organ or tissue is heavier or lighter than normal. However, it is difficult to measure organ weight in swine because of variable organ/body weight ratio and lack of well-established normographs unlike the case in laboratory animals. But some organs such as hearts endocrine glands, livers, kidneys can be weighted at necropsy. Hence, heavy implies something addedwhilelight implies something removed/taken away. Weight is most useful with lungs as it indicate whether blood and plasma resulting in congestion and edema is added to the lung or something is lost such as air sac collapse (referred as atelectasis). Hence, in case of lung, "The Bucket Test" is used to indirectly weigh the lungs in the following way. If the lung sinks in a bucket of water, something heavier than water is added OR, the air is removed (atelectasis is pretty common!) or both."

Assessment of the sound of a lesion is another special feature attributing the description of a lesion. Sound reference to how a lesion on organ or tissue resonances. Hence, lesion may produce crepitating, sloshing or hard sounds. Crepitating sound is the sound of popping air in case of for example emphysema, gas producing bacteria, normal lung. The absence such crepitating sound in lung indicate that the air sacs are collapsed (atelectasis). Sloshing sound is the sound of fluid splashing in case of Edema, ascites, pleural effusion and diarrhea. Hard type of sound sounds like a rock when banged on a hard surface. And this indicates sound of bone and mineralized matrix or calcifications of soft tissues.

Odor of a lesion is also another special feature of a given lesion which need to be considered during necropsy. This is because odor of a lesion may indicate the nature of the pathological process and its etiological basis, as it tells the smell. Hence, during necropsy, the person performing the necropsy need to bear in mind whether the lesion smell foul, ammonia, apple cider or no odor. Foul odor is rotting smell which indicate putrefactive necrosis, saprophytic agents or liquefactive necrosis. Ammonia like smelling of a lesion usually means uremia, excess blood urea nitrogen or urine accumulation in peritoneal cavity. Apple cider smell indicate gastric hemorrhage or swallowed blood. No odor which is very common indicate whether the lesion is many septic as well as aseptic processes.

J. Extent

Finally, one need to note the extent of the lesion to describe how much of the organ or tissue is affected. Because know the extent of the lesion on the organ or tissue is very helpful in making appropriate interpretations on the stage, severity of the pathological process. One measure of the severity and therefore the potential clinical significance of the gross lesions. Most important in lungs and kidneys where we have estimates of the physiologic reserve. The extent can be estimated in percentage of the total organ or tissue which is affected and potentially functionally compromised.

K. Chronicity of the lesions

It is subjectiveassessment of a lesions. This has to be noted while describing each though it is difficult to be precise and have a "real time" definition of chronic. Based on the stage of the chronicity of the lesions, they can be categorized into Acute, sunacute, chronic for lesion produced in seconds to hours, seconds to days, and weeks and above, respectively. Additionally, it can be also described as mixture of Acute and Chronic which may imply ongoing damage. The following are the gross hallmarks of chronicity. For instance, proliferation of cells takes time and thus evidence of cellular proliferation makes it likely the lesion is chronic. Deposition of stroma or extra cellular matrix show Fibrosis, hyperostosis. Larger size changes in organs either way (increased or decreased) imply a passage of time e.g. Hypertrophy, atrophy. Therefore, we need to consider "The Logic Test" by asking a the following question, "Is the lesion.... seconds, minutes, hours, days, weeks, months or years old"? And then, arrive at a logical range for the age of the lesion you observe.

L. Severity of the lesions

Severity of gross lesions is subjective assessment, sliding scale, relative, variable among pathologists. Often a 5 point scale used:

- Minimal
- Mild
- Moderate?
- Marked
- Severe

Not bad (Minimal, Mild)

Bad (Marked, Severe)

Step 1: Presence of abnormality: check presence of lesion

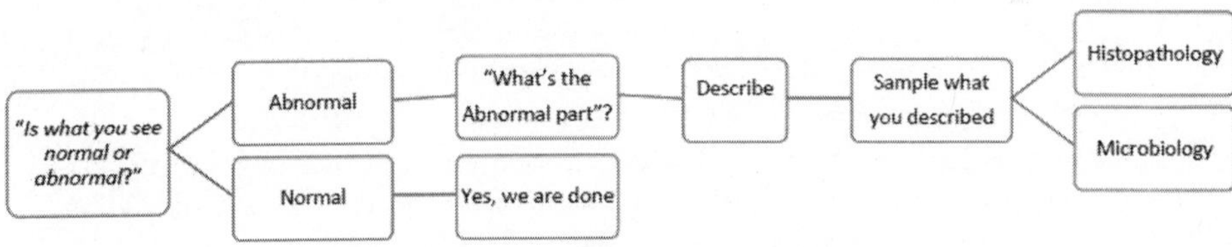

Step 2: Describe the abnormal part with respect to the above listed attributes which are appropriate. Not all the attributes will be relevant to every lesion. However, most can be described with respect to distribution, contour, color, size, consistency, extent of the organ affected and any special features unique to it. AA description doesn=t need to be a dissertation.

Step 3: Interpret a pathologic process from what you have described based upon what the attributes suggest. This is the fun part. It=s a chance to apply what you have learned and when done in conjunction with submitting samples to a pathologist, you get feedback about your interpretation.

Finally, as necropsy in this setting should be a descriptive exercise to document the gross findings, a permanent record of the ephemeral events in the necropsy will be created. Moreover, required samples for histopathology, microbiology, toxicity, serology, etc. will be collected.

28.5.2 Interpretation of the described gross lesions

Following the thorough and complete description and recording of each and every gross lesion as per the above attributions, careful interpretation of the described lesions will be made by the skillful pathologist. The interpretation of the lesions need to explain the cause of death or establish/confirm the presence of absence of a disease entity. The histopathology is a permanent record because the blocks and slides are often housed for long periods of time but the history, clinical findings and the gross pathology are not. These findings often provide a guide for what tissues to sample for histopathology culture etc. and should correlate with the histopathologic findings. The interpretation of the gross lesions intended to test the disease recognition skills of pathologist at the clinical, whole animal, organ and tissue level. They are all about interpretation, not description. You do the description subconsciously. Look at the lesion, collect the visual information, match the signalment given, interpret the lesions and answer the questions. Do not describe lesions!!! The value of a pathologist is partly determined by his/her ability to interpret and explain, generate and test hypotheses based upon what they see (King et al., 2014; Paul, 2008; Gramer et al., 2005).

For instance, one can learn how the following descried case is interpreted. Upon necropsy of a pig cadaver, the following were reported by a pathologist. The pig lungs were diffuse dark red, wet, heavy and fluid flowed freely from the cut surface and airwaysinterpreted to be pulmonary congestion and edema. There is a 3 cm white round mass in the liver which had a soft, amorphous white cut surface, spreadable with a butter knife, and a thick fibrous capsule interpreted to be an abscess. Both kidneys were diffuse, pale, wet and bulged on cut surface interpreted to be acute tubular necrosis or nephrosis. The brain contained miliary 1 mm flat red foci on the surfaceinterpreted to be petechiae, possibly DIC (disseminated in to circulation) or acute meningitis. There was an anterior-ventral distribution involving 40% of both lungs which were plum colored, had adherent fibrinous material on the pleura, were firm and upon cut surface contained pus in the airways interpreted to be fibrinopurulent bronchopneumonia. This interpretation of the pathologic process is summarized into a phrase or sentence called the morphologic diagnosis.This is the stock in trade of pathologists. It is used as a sort of short hand to document or denote pathologic processes. Skillful application of accurate morphologic diagnoses is most important to pathologists and much time is spent in training learning to do this properly. It is not necessarily important for clinicians to do this but accurate descriptions of what they observe is so the pathologist may formulate a presumptive morphologic diagnosis from the clinician's description which can then be verified from the histopathology.

Types of lesion Interpretation: The interpretation of the described lesions could be morphological diagnosis, based on naming of the disease or condition, based on naming of a related clinical or clinic-pathologic abnormality or etiological diagnosis.

Morphologic diagnosis is a phrase or short sentence summarizing the principal characteristic or dominant pathologic process present in the organ or tissue. It should include an organ and distribution modifier and a process. For example, one can interpreted a lesions as follows. Segmental renal cortical necrosis (infarct), bilaterally symmetrical hyperostotic maxillary fibrous osteodystrophy, diffuse granulomatous enteritis, osteochondritis, bilateral multinodular thyroid follicular adenomas, leukoencephalomalacia, serous atrophy of fat or lymphoma. In making morphological diagnosis, the carpenter test i.e. ask and answer the following question "Can you close your eyes and see what you said or wrote?" and by doing so, It is a good self-evaluation for clarity and completeness.

Interpretation based on the name the disease or conditionrefers to the medical or common usage term for the disease depicted in the image. For instance, many different regional names of diseases. Say for example, neoplasms which can be both Fibrous osteodystrophy, vesicular stomatitis, pyometra, palatoschisis, cyclopia. Sometimes morphological diagnosis and Name the Disease can be the same. For instance, leukoencephalomalacia, osteochondritis and etc. On the other hand, Naming of a Related Clinical or Clinicopathologic Abnormality is naming of a related clinical abnormality that is associated with the type of lesion or disease. The abnormality is hematologic, biochemical, clinical etc rather than an anatomic lesion. For example, pathological conditions diagnosis this way include; hypercalcemia, hypochloremia, hyperkalemia, polyuria/polydipsia, an etc.

Etiologic diagnosisis a word or phrase that captures a pathologic process with a reference of tissue and a cause or condition if possible. However, it is not commonly used anymore but seen occasionally. There are many different ways to formulate these and no one way is correct. This type of response to diagnosis frees you from making a formal anatomic morphologic diagnosis. There may be overlap with other forms of diagnosis. Etiologic diagnoses can be of widely varying specificity. For example, Cutaneous acariasis, Verminous arteritis, Intestinal histoplasmosis (protozoal enteritis), Toxic hepatopathy (hepatic mycotoxicosis), Proliferative and exudative interstitial pneumonia (pulmonary Toxoplasmosis), Protozoal myelitis (Spinal sarcocystosis) are types of etiological diagnosis.

28.6 Sampling and submission recommendations

Necropsy given a golden opportunity for pathologists, microbiologists, toxicologists or other experts working veterinary disease diagnosis to adequately collect all sort of samples from any organ or tissue for further laboratory tests. However, the quality of the samples collected during necropsy depends on how carefully are these samples collected. To proceed with careful collection of samples, availability of appropriate sampling material and preservative should be made sure before the commencing the necropsy. As it is economically and technically difficult to collect all type samples, there must prior plan on what samples need to be collected. The plan can be made before the necropsy based on the clinical findings of the case or can be decided based on the necropsy findings later during the necropsy. In the plan, the type of samples required and laboratory test expected to be performed to definitely diagnosis the case should be stated and communicated.

Example, there was case of porcine diarrhea in one month and older pigs and samples were collected during necropsy as follows. For this purpose, 3 euthanized pigs with typical signs, acutely affected and untreated were selected for necropsy. Necropsy was performed as above and the following fresh and fixed samples were carefully collected and submitted for histopathology (Table 1). Moreover, the samples obtained from individual pig separately were coded to be identified easily.

Table 1: Type and size of tissue samples collected and submitted for histopathology.

Porcine Diarrhea		
TISSUE/SAMPLE	FRESH (chilled – not frozen)	FIXED (10% buffered formalin)
Serum	5 ml	
Brain	Cut brain in half longitudinally, slightly off the midline. Submit larger half fresh/chilled.	Fix the smaller half in formalin.
Tonsil	½	½
Lung	5 X 5 X 5 cm piece	2 X 2 X 1 cm
Liver	8 X 8 X 4 cm piece	2 X 2 X 0.5 cm
Kidney	Half of a kidney	0.5 cm slice, including cortex and medulla.
Spleen	10 cm piece	1 cm piece
Jejunum	15 cm segment	2 sections, 2 cm long, unopened
Ileum	15 cm segment	2 sections, 2 cm long, unopened
Mesenteric lymph node	Entire lymph node	1 cm thickness piece
Spiral Colon	2 10 cm segments (bagged separately from small intestine)	2 sections, 2 cm long, unopened
Fluid contents from cecum or colon	10 ml in leakproof container	

Chapter 29

Record Keeping in Swine Production

—Dr. Kiros Abebe & Mr.Hailay Kidanu

Record keeping is an important component of livestock business management. Without record maintenance, it is difficult for the farmers to memorize all expenses and activities while making decisions regarding their farm practices. Thus, recording of performance of the animals, economic development, or any activity of the farmer or veterinarian can help us to take good decisions and to keep track of activities, production and important events on a farm.

29.1 Advantages of Record Keeping at Farm

- It improve overall efficiency and to determine profitability.
- It provides the basis for evaluation of animals from past records to decide to select or cull the animals.
- It also helps in preparing pedigree and history record of animals.
- It produce end data to describe production and reproduction levels, economics of production, feed stock and feeding in animals, growth performance of animals.
- It helps in assessing the past records and designing better breeding plans to check inbreeding, selecting superior parents and helps in better replacement and culling practices.
- It helps to formulate economic feeding strategies for optimal productions.
- It helps to formulate precautionary measures like vaccination, deworming etc. as per disease record.
- For fixing proper prices of animal for purchase and sale.
- It determines the income and expenditure.
- Helps in estimating the cost of pork production.
- Helpful in comparing the efficiency of labour and herd with other farms.

- To compare the herd performances in different years to determine the amount of profit/loss each year and setting future goals/directions for the farm.

29.2 Types of Records to be Maintained at a Swine Farm

Kinds of Records

The major records maintained in tropical farms are: Individual pig register, Breeding register, Litter record, Farrowing register, ledger, Health register, Daily feed register, Cash book, purchase book, Store stock book, Bill payable book, Inventory register, Weight register, Feed order book, Attendance/pay register etc.

Some of the most common records are described below. These are individual pig register, breeding register, farrowing record, feeding register, litter record, inventory record.

1. Individual pig register: This register records the details of the individual animals at the farm along with their identification number, sex, number of teats, birth weight, coat color, off color mark, weaning weight (kg.) at 56 days, defects / remarks (table 28.1).

Table 28.1: Individual pig register

Pig no.	Sex	Number of teats	Birth weight	Coat color	Off color mark	Weaning weight (kg.) at 56 days	Defects / remarks

2. Breeding register: This register maintains the details of breeding practices in the farm such as sow number, date of farrowing, date of first and last farrowing, services along with the boar number, date of successful service, expected date of farrowing etc (table 28.2).

Table 28.2: Breeding register

No. of sows	Date		No. of farrowing completed	Date of last farrowing	Boar assigned	Date of service	Date of farrow
	Birth	First farrowing					

3. Farrowing record: This register maintains the records of farrowing that take place in the farm. It maintains sow number, farrowing date, litter size and their sex, number of dead piglets and the total number of piglets raised (table 28.3).

Table 28.3: Farrowing register

No. of sow	Farrowing date	No. of piglet born	No. of pigs born			Total no. of pig raised
			Live		Dead	
			Male	Female		

4. Feeding register for the month ………………………………..

This register records the amount concentrate, dry fodder, green fodder and other feeds given to the animals (table 28.4).

Table 28.4: Feeding register

Date	Feed amount (BF)	Feed purchased	Total feed in stock	No. of pigs	Feed issued (Kg.)	Balance of feed (CF)

5. Inventory register:

Table 28.5: Inventory register

Sl. No.	Animal no.	Sex	Class	Birth date	Age	Stock value	Depreciation	Present value

6. Health Record: This register maintains the record of the diseased animals along with vaccination and deworming given.

Date of Hog cholera vaccination: ______________

Date of Erysipelas vaccination: ________________

Piglet record: Number born (total): ____________

Alive: ____________; Males: ______________; Females: _________________

Date of deworming: _________________________

Mummies: ______________; Males: _______________; Females: ____________

Pig weaned: _______________; Males: ____________; Females: _____________

7. Litter records:

Litter number: Breed: __________

Dam record:

Number / name: _____________________ Sire:

Birth date: ___________________________ Dam:

Number of carcass: _________________ Average back fat: _________ cm^2

Sows: ___________ Litter I, II, III etc.) Loin eye: ________ cm^2;

Loin length: _______ cm^2

Sire record:

Number / name: _____________________ Sire:

Birth date: ___________________________ Dam:

Number of carcass: _________________ Average back fat: _________ cm^2

Sows: ___________ Litter I, II, III etc.) Loin eye: ________ cm^2;

Loin length: _______ cm^2

❑❑❑

Chapter 30

Disinfection of Swine Barns

— Dr. Muuz Gebru & Dr. Endale Balcha

Cleaning meant for removal of dirt, faecal matter, leftover feed, slurry and other organic and inorganic impurities from the surface using water, soap, detergents or physically. Sanitizing lowers the microbial number from the surface while disinfection kill germs on surface or objects. The five basic steps of cleaning and disinfection are remove organic matter (bedding, feed residue dried faeces, slurry and dust etc. with water), use of detergent followed by cleaning, drying and finally disinfection. Disinfectants have two prime functions. First to prevent infectious agents gaining access to the farm and second equally important to control those organisms already on the farm and that persist in large numbers in the environment.

Disinfectants are chemical agent applied to inanimate objects that kill both harmless and disease producing organisms. They act either as bacterial poisons, coagulate bacterial protein or act as oxidising or reducing agents. Sanitizers are chemical agents that reduces the bacterial, fungal, or viral population without killing the microorganism when applied to inanimate objects. Antiseptics normally prevent bacterial multiplication and are used for cleaning skin or wounds. Some disinfectants in a more dilute form may act as antiseptics. Detergentsare chemical agents that contains both cleansers and solvents and are added to water in order to reduce surface tension and to increase penetrating ability of water. This allows more organic matter (dirt) to be removed from surfaces.

30.1 Characteristics of an Ideal Disinfectant:

- Non-irritating and nontoxic to man and animals.
- Noncorrosive and non-staining to equipment and surfaces.
- Broad spectrum effectiveness against various infectious agents.

- No residue in meat.
- Cheaper and easily available
- Residual effect.
- Capability to penetrate, preferably with a detergent action.
- Stable when diluted.
- Unaffected by environmental factors: organic matter, dirt, dust, soaps or detergents, pH, temperature, and relative humidity.
- Readily soluble in hard water.

Efficacy of Disinfectants is affected by temperature, presence of organic matter, pH, concentration of disinfectant etc. the efficacy of chlorine and iodine decreases above 110 F. Iodophors and chlorine compounds are not effective when organic matter (like dirt, dust, manure, and left feed) is present. Synthetic phenols, and cresylic acids are more effective in disinfecting surfaces covered with organic matter. Iodophors, chlorine, and phenols are more effective at a low pH while quaternary ammonium compounds are more active at a high pH.

30.2 Types of Disinfectant Used

Phenolic compounds: They have a wide range of antimicrobial activity. Usually effective in the present of organic matter. They are non-corrosive to metal but they can cause damage to plastic and rubber compounds. Their activity persists for a long period of time. They are used widely on concrete floor and for vehicle dips due to its cheaper price. The efficacy is good against bacteria but not so good against viruses or spore producing bacteria.

Iodophors: They are safe and almost odourless. Iodophors are more effective against viruses and bacteria. They ideal for disinfecting equipment and clean surfaces but also used in foot baths. They are moderately active in the present of organic matter. They are comparatively expensive. They are also used as water sanitizer (effective levels at 12.5-25 ppm.).

Chlorine: They are cheaper and widely used disinfectant. The presence of organic matter and sunlight reduces its disinfecting properties. They are corrosive to some surfaces and have very rapid action against most microorganisms. As a water sanitizer, they are effective at 3-10 ppm.

Quaternary Ammonium Compounds (QAC): They have good bactericidal, viricidal and fungicidal activity and are commonly used for disinfecting meat-packing and food-handling equipment. They are not sporicidal. The efficacy decrease in the presence of organic matter and detergents.

Potassium monopersulfate (Tade name Vircon): It has wide spectrum of viricidal, bactericidal, and fungicidal activity. The surfactant and organic acid components enhance this affect.

Saponated Solution of Cresol: It contain soap and are more effective in hot solutions. They are effective on surfaces with minimal organic matter present.

Table 1. Characteristics of Some Common Disinfectants

Characteristics	*Chlorine*	*Iodine*	*Quaternary Ammonium*	*Phenol*	*Cresol*
Residual	-	+/-	+	slight	+
Corrosive	+	+/-	-	slight	+
Irritating	+	+/-	-	+	+
Active in Organic Matter	-	-	+	+	+
Staining	+	+/-	-	-	+
Volatile	+	+/-	+	-	-
Expense	low	moderate	moderate	moderate	high

Table 2: Information About Common Disinfectants

Chemical compound	*Gram + Bacteria*	*Gran - Bacteria*	*Fungi*	*Virus*	*Best pH range for activity*	*Activity when organic matter present*	*Common uses*
Chlorhexidene	Some activity	Some activity	Some activity	Most	Wide range	Good	Equipment / Premises / Footbaths
Formaldehyde and aldehydes	++	++	++	++	Wide range	Good	Equipment / Premises / Footbaths
Chlorine Chloramines	++	++	++	Some activity	Acid	Very poor	Clean surfaces/ Equipment
Iodophors	++	++	++	Some activity	Acid	Fair to poor	Clean surfaces/ Equipment
Sodium hydroxide	++	++	++	++	Alkaline	Good	Premises
Quaternary ammoniums	++	+	Some activity	Some activity	Alkaline	Fair	Clean surfaces/ Equipment
Phenols	++	++	Some activity	Some activity	Acid	+Good	Equipment / Premises / Footbaths

Chapter 31

Economics of Setting up of a Pig Rearing Farm

—Dr. Etsay Kebede

31.1 General consideration for establishment of farm

For establishment of 30 sows and 3 boar's farm, the following consideration are assumed:

Space requirement:

- **Boar:** Covered floor area per boar (m^2): 6.25-7.5; open area per boar (m^2): 8.8-12.0
- **Farrowing:** Covered floor area per boar (m^2): 7.5-9.0; open area per boar (m^2): 8.8-12.0
- **Weaner:** Covered floor area per boar (m^2): 0.95-1.8; open area per boar (m^2): 8.8-12.0
- **Dry sow:** Covered floor area per boar (m^2): 1.8-2.7; open area per boar (m^2): 1.5-1.8

Other assumptions:

- Marketable age of piglets: 180 days
- Litter size: 10
- Mortality: 10%
- Viable litter size: 9
- Weight at marketable age: 75 kg
- Number of farrowing per year: 2
- Insurance Coverage: 6.5 % of total purchase cost of parent stock

Scheme for establishment of 30+3 pig unit

I. Capital expenditure

- Purchase of 30 gilt: **a**
- Purchase of 3 male Weaner for Breeding Boar: **b**
- Farm construction: **c**
- Total = **a + b + c = A**

II. Recurring expenditure

- Concentrate (grower) for 6 month @ 1.5kg/day/animal 1.5 30 6 30 = 8,100 kg: **d**
- Concentrate (breeder Ration) 2kg 5 30days 6 months 30 pigs = 10,800 kgs: **e**
- Medicine and vaccines: **f**
- Insurance Coverage 6.5 % of total purchase cost of parent stock: **g**
- Transportation cost: **h**
- Unskilled Labour Cost – 2 Nos. for 1 year: **i**
- Equipments: **j**
- Biosecurity and water: **k**
- Miscellaneous: **l**
- **Total = d + e + f + g + h + i+ j + k + l = B**

III. Financial Arrangement

Total expenditure for 30 Sows + 3 Breeding Boars = A + B = C

III. Expected return:

Particulars	*1st year*	*2nd year*	*3rd year*	*4th year*
Total piglets of both sex	270	540	540	540
• Male piglets	135	135	135	135
• Female piglets	135	135	135	135
Income generation				
Sale of male piglets @ 6 months age	w_1	w_2	w_3	w_4
Sale of female piglets @ 6 months age	x_1	x_2	x_3	x_4
Sale of Gunny Bag	y_1	y_2	y_3	y_4
Sale of manure	z_1	z_2	z_3	z_4
Total	$w_1+x_1+y_1+z_1 = P_1$	$w_2+x_2+y_2+z_2 = P_2$	$w_3+x_3+y_3+z_3 = P_3$	$w_4+x_4+y_4+z_4 = P_4$

Annual expenditure

Concentrate (grower)	a_1	a_2	a_3	a_4
Concentrate (breeder Ration)	b_1	b_2	b_3	b_4
Medicine and vaccines	c_1	c_2	c_3	c_4
Insurance Coverage	d_1	d_2	d_3	d_4
Transportation cost	e_1	e_2	e_3	e_4
Labour Cost	f_1	f_2	f_3	f_4
Equipments	g_1	g_2	g_3	g_4
Biosecurity and water	h_1	h_2	h_3	h_4
Miscellaneous	i_1	i_2	i_3	i_4
	$a_1 + b_1 + c_1 + d_1 + e_1 + f_1 + g_1 + h_1 + i_1 = Q_1$	$a_2 + b_2 + c_2 + d_2 + e_2 + f_2 + g_2 + h_2 + i_2 = Q_2$	$a_3 + b_3 + c_3 + d_3 + e_3 + f_3 + g_3 + h_3 + i_3 = Q_3$	$a_4 + b_4 + c_4 + d_4 + e_4 + f_4 + g_4 + h_4 + i_4 = Q_4$

Income per annum

	1st year	2nd year	3rd year	4th year
Income per annum	P1 - Q1	P2 – Q2	P3 – Q3	P4 – Q4

❑❑❑

Chapter 32

Terms Used in Swine Industry

—Dr. Niraj Kumar

- **Abattoir:** A slaughterhouse.
- **Abortion:** The observed production of foetuses between services and up to, and including, the 109th day of pregnancy.
- **Age of gilts mated (average):** The total age in days of gilts, at mating, divided by the number of gilts (approximately 7 to 8 months).
- **Anthelmintic:** A drug treatment used to expel parasitic worms. An example of a typical anthelmintic is Ivomectin.
- **Ark:** A low semi-circular field-shelter for pigs.
- **Artificial insemination:** The process of breeding a sow by using semen extracted from a boar instead of natural mating. This is a good way to add better genetics to a herd without raising multiple boars.
- **Backfatter:** Culled breeding pig sold for meat; usually refers specifically to a culled sow, but is sometimes used in reference to boars.
- **Baconer:** A pig being reared for bacon rather than pork, and which will be slaughtered at 80kg to 100kg live weight which it attains at about 8 - 10 months of age.
- **Barrow:** Male pig castrated before puberty.
- **Belly:** The underside of a pig.
- **Blind Teat:** An irregular teat that is sometimes removed to prevent piglets from attempting to nurse on a useless teat.
- **Boar:** An uncastrated male pig over six months old (breeding age).
- **Body Capacity:** This term describes the shape of a pig in relation to growth, health, feed conversion, and the quality potential of the carcass.

- **Bone:** This describes the diameter of the bone in the legs, jaw and the width of the head. Good bone is important for determining how well the pig will carry its weight.
- **Breeding Herd:** Consists of gilts, sows, and boars. Including replacement gilts that are used to maintain a herd of pigs.
- **Bulk:** Refers to a pig's diet. Bulk is the fibre added either separately or mixed in the pigs feed.
- **Butcher Hog:** A butcher hog, also known as a market hog, is a pig that weighs between 220 and 260 pounds, is approximately 6 months old, and was raised to for slaughter.
- **Carcass:** The carcass is the body of a pig after it has been dressed out (butchered).
- **Castration:** To sterilize a male pig by removing the testicles.
- **Chitterlings:** The small intestines of a pig. Can be prepared for consumption.
- **Colostrum:** First milk produced by the sow; it provides immunity to the baby pigs for the first few weeks.
- **Conception rate:** The number of sows that conceive to service expressed as a percentage of these services. Conception is assumed by non-return to oestrous 21 days after service, or identified by pregnancy diagnosis at about 30 days post-service. These measures are not precise and the term 'conception rate' is therefore of limited use.
- **Condition scoring:** A method of estimating the fat cover on sows so that feeding levels can be determined.
- **Cracklings:** Cracklings are the by-product of rendering lard. They are pieces of skin and meat that were browned. Also referred to as pork rinds.
- **Creep Feed:** Creep feed is a starter ration for piglets. It is high in protein, usually from sugar and milk proteins for high energy.
- **Creep feeder:** Area accessible to small pigs but not their dams, in which a high protein supplement is provided.
- **Cross Breeding:** Cross breeding is a method used to maximize the quality traits of different breeds into a faster growing market hog.
- **Cross-fostering:** A management practice involving fostering piglets to benefit sows and litters.
- **Cull sow:** Full-grown female sold for slaughter. Usually showing poor physical characteristics that make her undesirable for breeding.
- **Culled sow or boar:** Any live sow or boar removed from the breeding unit.
- **Culling percentage** = (Total number of sows and boars sold and transferred x 100)/ average number of sows (see 'herd size') and boars.
- **Culling:** This is the process of removing any undesirable animals from the herd normally for health or performance issues.

- **Cuts:** The end products of pork after the butchering process is complete. Usually packaged into individual serving sizes.
- **Daily dressed weight gain (individual):** The dressed weight of the pig divided by the number of days from birth, when leaving the farm, expressed in grams per day.
- **Daily live weight gain (group average):** The total live weight gain of pigs divided by the total number of pig days, expressed in grams per day.
- **Daily live weight gain (individual):** The total live weight gain of the pig, for a specified period, divided by the number of days over the same given period, expressed in grams per day e.g. 500 grams/day (0 to 90 kg), 700 grams/day (40 to 90 kg).
- **Dam:** The female parent.
- **Dark firm and dry pork (DFD):** Meat in which muscles are dark in colour, may be sticky and holds water well.
- **Dewclaw:** The small appendage just above the hoof on the posterior side.
- **Dressed weight or Hanging weight:** The weight of a pig carcass after it has been gutted and prepped for butchering.
- **Dressing percent:** Percentage of the butchered carcass that is usable, compared to live weight.
- **Drift:** A group of young pigs.
- **Drove:** A herd or group of pigs.
- **Empty days (herd average):** (365 herd farrowing index) - (herd lactation length + 114)
- **Empty days:** The number of days between weaning or sows initial service and effective service or removal from the breeding herd.
- **Estrus:** When a female animal is in heat and ready to mate.
- **Failure to farrow:** Sow not farrowed by 120 days after presumed effective service.
- **Farrow to Finish:** This means raising the pig from birth to butchering size.
- **Farrowing index (herd) or litters per sow per year:** The number of farrowings taking place in a given period, expressed on an annual basis, divided by the average number of sows in the herd during the period when those sows were mated.
- **Farrowing interval:** The number of days from one farrowing to the next farrowing.
- **Farrowing rate:** The number of sows that farrow to a given number of services expressed as a percentage.
- **Farrowing:** Birth of a littler of piglets.
- **Feed conversion ratios:** The total weight of air-dry food consumed by a pig or pigs divided by its/their live weight (or dead weight) gain over a given period. This measure can be calculated over different periods of the pig's life or as an average over the whole herd by the formula.

- **Feed Efficiency:** The amount of feed needed for a pig to gain one pound of weight. This is an important factor when choosing pigs for farrow to finish.
- **Feeder pig:** A weaned gilt or barrow weighing between 18 kg (40 lb) and 37 kg (82 lb) at 6 to 8 weeks of age that is sold to be finished for slaughter.
- **Finisher:** A grower pig over 70 kg (150 lb) of live weight.
- **Finishing:** Feeding a pig out to reach market weight.
- **Fitting:** Getting a pig ready for a show or exhibit.
- **Flush feed:** Increase feed to stimulate ovulation in females.
- **Forage:** When pigs attain their own food by searching their environment.
- **Fostering:** The act of transferring a sucker or suckers from one sow to another.
- **Frame:** The skeletal system of a pig. Large frames are desirable in pigs. Also relevant to bone.
- **Full Feed:** Animals are allowed to eat as much as they will clean up; feed is available at all times.
- **Full-term empty:** Sows that go full-term, presumed pregnant, and do not farrow.
- **Gestation Period:** Length of pregnancy. In pigs it is 114 days.
- **Gilt:** Young female not yet mated, or not yet farrowed, or after only one litter.
- **Hand Mating:** It refers to the practice of placing a boar in a pen with only one sow or gilt.
- **Herd:** A group of pigs, or all the pigs on a farm or in a region.
- **Heritage breed:** The pedigree of a purebred animal that descends from a time before industrial farming.
- **Heterosis:** The process of cross-breeding pigs to produce more favourable breed traits such as litter size, conception rate, piglet survival rate and growth.
- **Hock:** The back leg joint.
- **Hog or swine:** It represent species as a whole and synonym for pig. Swine is used as singular as well as plural.
- **Hogging Down:** Letting pigs into a crop field to clean up or harvest the crop.
- **Hogging:** Describes the behaviour of a sow when on heat (during oestrous).
- **In pig:** When a sow is pregnant she is in pig.
- **Inbreeding:** This is the mating of two animals that are closely related in order to bring out the good traits. This doesn't always work as hoped. Farmers call it Line breeding when it works and Inbreeding when it doesn't.
- **Jowl:** The underside of a pig's neck.

- **Lactation:** This is the time when a sow is producing milk and feeding piglets.
- **Lard:** Lard is rendered pork fat. There are many uses for lard besides cooking.
- **Leg:** The leg of a pig from which ham is derived.
- **Libido:** When a sow is ready for breeding she will show sexual interest.
- **Limit Feeding:** This is simply restricting the feed of sows and boars alike to avoid obesity and lengthen the time they pigs will be able to produce.
- **Line Breeding:** Repeatedly breeding a specific pig to generate offspring with specific traits. Breeding sibling to sibling or parent to offspring. Also called inbreeding.
- **Line:** A specific bloodline that can be traced to a specific animal or family group.
- **Litter scatter:** An index indicating herds with numbers of pigs born per litter to one standard deviation above and below an average litter size within any specified period.
- **Litter weight variability:** The range of weights at birth.
- **Litter:** A group of piglets born to a single sow.
- **Loin:** The muscles on either side of the spine which produces pork tenderloins.
- **Maintenance:** The requirements of the animal for nutrients for the continuity of vital processes, within the body, including the replacements of obligatory losses in faeces, urine and skin, are met, so that the net gain or loss of nutrients and other tissue substances by the animal as a whole is zero.
- **Mash:** Feed that has been ground. Usually fed to young pigs and sick pigs.
- **Meal:** Feed ground to a fine texture like cornmeal.
- **Niddle or pin teeth:** These are the two teeth on either side of the jaw that look like canine teeth. They are extremely sharp and can damage a sows teats. Many commercial farms clip the needle teeth at birth. They are also called eye teeth or wolf teeth.
- **Offal:** Often referred to as animal waste, offal are actually the internal organs of a butchered pig.
- **Open:** This term refers to a gilt or so that did not conceive at breeding or may have absorbed the pregnancy.
- **Orphan piglet:** Feeding piglets whose mother does not produce enough milk or dies, the piglet should give to another sow which farrowed or gave birth.
- **Overlaying:** When a sow crushes and kills her piglets by laying on them which results in crushing. This is quite common and results in many losses for pig farmers.

- **Parity:** The number of litters a sow has carried (including current pregnancy), e.g. a second parity sow is in pig with or suckling her second litter.
- **Pastern:** The bone that connects the hoof and leg joints.
- **Pig Boards:** They are made from plastic and plywood, between 30 and 40 inches high and have hand holes cut in them. Pig boards are used to guide pigs when they are being moved. See also "hurdle".
- **Piglet:** Unweaned young pig or any immature pig or newly borne.
- **Pig-shed:** A larger pig-house.
- **Porker:** A pig reared to pork weight, normally about 60kg live weight, rather than to bacon weight. Usually achieved between four to six months of age, depending on breed.
- **Premix:** This is a mineral pack that feed producers use to create a balanced diet in swine feed.
- **Primal Cuts:** This refers to large cuts during butchering such as half a pig or a quarter of the carcass.
- **Probiotics:** These are beneficial organisms used to aid sick or recovering animals. Probiotics are also used to help stimulate nutrient absorption.
- **Processing:** Preparing a slaughtered animal for packaging or storage.
- **Prolificacy:** Refers to the number of piglets produced by a sow or boar. Boars and sows that are not prolific, are culled.
- **Purebred:** Pigs that have been bred to members of their own breed and usually have pedigrees to prove their lineage.
- **Ration (scale feeding):** Refers to the weight of complete diet offered daily and is not confined to energy intake; it may be given either in a single portion or in a number of portions each day. When the level of feeding is increased, daily intakes of all nutrients are thus increased.
- **Rear flank:** Located between the ribs and stifle.
- **Render:** Cooking down the fat remove impurities and moisture prior to storing.
- **Restricted feeding:** Feeding systems where the feed is rationed to an individual pig or group of pigs and is under the daily control of the person feeding the pigs. Amounts given are usually restricted to less than the pigs' maximum voluntary intake at each feed and are most commonly given once or divided equally into a number of portions, each day. The feed may be given either wet or dry. Same as controlled feeding.
- **Return to service:** A sow re-served after a previous unsuccessful service.
- **Ring:** Placing a metal ring in a hog's snout to keep them from rooting.
- **Rooting:** When pigs dig up the earth with their noses in search of food.
- **Rotational grazing:** The practice of moving pigs from one pasture to another to maximize feeding, minimize parasites, and/or hog down a pasture.

- **Rump:** The area on a pig's back just above its tail.
- **Runt:** An unusually small and weak piglet, often one in a litter.
- **Scours:** Diarrhoea. Severe scours can cause death.
- **Service index:** The number of services taking place in one year divided by the average herd size.
- **Service:** The introduction of semen into the uterus of a sow or gilt. This can be natural (done by a boar) or by artificial insemination.
- **Settle:** After a sow or gilt has taken to a pregnancy she is considered settled.
- **Shoat:** A young pig that has not yet reached 120 pounds.
- **Snout:** A pig's nose.
- **Soft Pork:** Butchered pork that remains oily, flabby, and soft even after chilling. This meat is considered undesirable.
- **Sounder:** A small group of pigs (or wild boar) foraging in woodland.
- **Sow to boar ratio:** The ratio of sows to boars as defined. This must take into account the non-working boar.
- **Sow:** Breeding female after first litter.
- **Stag:** A male pig that was castrated after reaching sexual maturity.
- Standing Heat: When a sow or gilt is ready to be serviced. She will acquirean rigid posture when pressure is applied on her back.
- **Stifle:** The knee joint in the hind leg.
- **Sty:** A small pig-house, usually with an outdoor run or a pig confinement.
- **Sucker/ Suckling pig:** A pig between birth and weaning or a piglet (mostly stay around their parents) slaughtered for its tender meat.
- **Team or Passel:** A group of hogs.
- **Top Dress:** Manually adding supplements to a hogs feed.
- **Trotters:** The hooves of pigs (they have four hoofed toes on each foot, walking mainly on the larger central two).
- **Underline:** Commonly used to describe the underside or belly of a sow. This term is used to evaluate teat placement on the underline for adequate milk production and ability to feed piglets. It is also used to evaluate the penis placement and sheath of a boar.
- **Vulva:** The exposed portion of a sows genitals. Changes in the vulva are useful in determining heat or preparation for farrowing in a sow or gilt.
- **Wallow:** A muddy puddle pigs use to cool their body temperature in hot weather.
- **Weaner:** A piglet separated from its mother and eating only solid food. Weaning can take place anytime between three to eight weeks of age. In tropics, weaning takes place usually at 8 weeks of age.
- **Weaning:Removing young from their mother.** Weaning can take place anywhere from 3 to 8 weeks depending on the farmers growing system.

- **Weanling:** A piglet recently removed from the sow and typically weighing between 25 and 40 pounds.
- **Yield:** Percentage of the carcass in the four lean cuts: ham, loin, picnic and Boston butt.

❑❑❑

References

Adzitey, F. 2011. Effect of pre-slaughter animal handling on carcass and meat quality, International Food Research Journal 18: 485-491

AHDB. 2008. Structure of the UK Pig Industry. A survey of loose housed systems by Analysis Group. Agriculture and Horticulture Development Board

AHDB. 2016. Pig holdings in the UK. Agriculture and Horticulture Development Board Available from: www.pork.ahdb.org.uk/prices-stats/industry-structure/pig-holdings-in-the-uk

Álvarez, D., Garrido, M.D. and Bañón, S. 2009. Influence of Pre-Slaughter Process on Pork Quality: An Overview, Food Reviews International, 25:3, 233-250, DOI:10.1080/87559120902956216

Andrzej P. and Tomasz F. 2006. Critical points in the development of pork quality – a review, polish journal of food and nutrition sciences, 2006, 15/56 (3): 249–256

Baker, Meelee, and Robert E. Mikesell. 1996. Animal Science Biology and Technology. Danville, Ill.: Interstate Publishers, Inc.

Banerjee, G. C. 2010. A Textbook of Animal Husbandry, Oxford and IBH Publishing Co. Pvt. Ltd., New Delhi, India, 8th edition.

Baxter, S. 1984. Intensive Pig Production: Environmental Management and Design. Granada, New York, NY.

Becerril-Herrera, M., Alonso-Spilsbury, M., Lemus-Flores, C., Guerrero-Legarreta, I., Olmos-Hernández, A., Ramírez-Necoechea, R. and Mota-Rojas, D. 2009. CO2 stunning may compromise swine welfare compared with electrical stunning, Meat Science 81: 233–237

Becker, H. Neil, George W. Meyerholz, and Jack M. Gaskin. "Selection and Use of Disinfectants in Disease Prevention." Pork Industry Handbook. PIH-80. Lafayette, Indiana.

Beltrán-Alcrudo, D., Arias, M., Gallardo, C., Kramer, S. & Penrith, M.L. (2017). African swine fever: detection and diagnosis. A manual for veterinarians. FAO Animal Production and Health Manual No. 19. Rome. Food and Agriculture Organization of the United Nations (FAO). 88 pages.

Benjamin, N. 2018. Tips for proper selection of cleaning, disinfection products, The Pig Site, https://pighealthtoday.com/tips-for-proper-selection-of-cleaning-disinfection-products/

Boggs, Donald L., and Robert A. Merkel. 1993. Live Animal Carcass Evaluation and Selection Manual. 4th ed. Dubuque: Kendall/Hunt Publishing Company.

Booth, C.M. 2018. Should you rotate disinfectants? Industry experts weigh in. Pharmaceutical ONLINE, https://www.pharmaceuticalonline.com/doc/should-you-rotate-disinfectants-industry-experts-weigh-in-0001.

Bowman A.S et al. 2015. Effects of disinfection on the molecular detection of porcine epidemic diarrhea virus. Veterinary Microbiology 179:213-8.

Bracke, M.B.M. 2011. "Review of wallowing in pigs: description of the behaviour and its motivational basis". Applied Animal Behaviour Science. 132 (1–2): 1–13.

Bruins, G. and Dyer, J.A. 1995. Environmental considerations of disinfectants used in agriculture, Rev.Sci.Tech.Off.Int.Epiz.14:81-94.

Castren, H.; Algers, B.; Jensen, P.; Saloniemi, H. 1989. "Suckling behaviour and milk consumption in new-born piglets as a response to sow grunting". Applied Animal Behaviour Science. 24 (3): 227–238.

Chauhan, R.S. and D. Chandra, 2007. Necropsy and Histopathological examination techniques. Veterinary Laboratory Diagnosis, 2nd ed., Centre for Animal Disease Research and Diagnosis, Indian Veterinary Research Institute. International Distributing Co., pp: 243-269.

Chulayo, A.Y. and Muchenje V. 2015. A balanced perspective on animal welfare for improved meat and meat products. South Africa Journal of Animal Science 45 (5): 452-469.

obanovi , N., Boškovi , M., Vasilev, D., Dimitrijevi , M., Parunovi , N., Djordjevi J. and Karabasi, N. 2016. Effects of various pre-slaughter conditions on pig carcasses and meat quality in a low-input slaughter facility, South African Journal of Animal Science, 46 (4)

Cutler, R., J. P. Hurtgen and A. D. Leman. 1981. "Reproductive System", Diseases of Swine. Ames, Iowa: Iowa State University Press, pp. 96-129.

Cutler, R., J. P. Hurtgen, and A. D. Leman. 1986. Diseases of Swine, 6th Edition. Ames, Iowa: Iowa State University Press.

Czy ak-Runowska, G., Wojtczak, J., Łyczy ski, A., Wójtowski, J., Markiewicz-K szycka, M., Stanisławski, D. and Babicz, M. 2015. Meat quality of crossbred porkers without the gene RYR1T Depending on slaughter weight. Asian Australas Journal of Animal Science, 28 (3): 398-404.

Devendra, C. and M.F. Fuller. 1979. Pig Production in the Tropics. Oxford, Great Britain: Oxford University Press.

Devendra, C., Thomas D., Jabbar M. A. and Kudo H. 1997. Improvement of Livestock Production in Crop-Animal System in Rain fed Agro ecological Zones of South-East Asia; 116 pp., ILRI (International Livestock Research Institute), Nairobi, Kenya. ISBN: 92-9146-031-1.

Edwards, S. 2011. Pigs. Management and welfare of farmed animals. UFAW Farm Handbook.

Ensminger, M. E. 1992. Stockman's Handbook Digest. Danville, Ill.: Interstate Publishers, Inc.

FAO. (2013). Food Outlook Biannual Report on Global Food Markets. ISSN: 0251-1959. http://www.fao.org/3/a-I5703E.pdf.

FAOSTAT, 2018. Food and Agriculture Organization of the United Nations. http://www.fao.org/faostat/en/#data/QA

FAOSTAT. 2013. Food and Agriculture Organisation of the United Nations Statistics Division. Faostat3/fao.org

Farmer, C. 2015. The gestating and lactating sow. The Netherlands: Wageningen Academic Publishers. ISBN 9789086868032. OCLC 899008362

FAWC. 2015. Opinion on Free Farrowing Systems. Farm Animal Welfare Council www.gov.uk/government/uploads/system/uploads/attachment_data/file/478588...

Gene A. Futrell, Iowa State University; Allan G. Mueller, University of Illinois; Glenn Grimes 2017. Understanding Hog Production and Price Cycles. Home resources areas eXTENSION.ORG accessed Nov 27/2017.

Gillespie, J.R. 1997. Animal Science. An International Thomson Publishing company ITP. Delmar Publishers.

Gillespie, James R. 1997. Modern Livestock and Poultry Production. 5th ed. Albany: Delmar.

Gispert, M., Angels Oliver, M., Velarde, A., Suarez, P., Pérez, J., Font i Furnols, M., 2010. Carcass and meat quality characteristics of immunocastrated male, surgically castrated male, entire male and female pigs. Meat Sci. 85, 664-670.

Giuffra, E; Kijas, JM; Amarger, V; Carlborg, O; Jeon, JT; Andersson, L. 2000. "The origin of the domestic pig: independent domestication and subsequent introgression". Genetics. 154 (4): 1785–91.

Grandin, T., K. Ernst, D. Ernst, and J. J. McGlone. 1989. Handling hogs. PIH-116, Pork industry handbook. Cooperative Extension Service, Purdue University, West Lafayette, IN.

Guardia M.D., Estany, J. Balasch, S., Oliver, M.A., Gispert, M. and Diestre A. 2004. Risk assessment of PSE condition due to pre-slaughter conditions and RYR1 gene in pigs, Meat Science 67: 471–478

Guide to Environmental Quality in Pork Production. Des Moines: National Pork Producers Council, 1993.

Harris D. L.; Multi-Site Pig Production; 2000, 280 pp., Iowa state University Press, Iowa, USA. ISBN: 813826993.

Herrick, John B. 1986. Immunology and Swine Production. Annual Health and Nutrition.

Holness, D. H; Pigs; Vol. 132, 1991, 150 pp., Macmillan Press Ltd., Basingstoke, UK. ISBN: 0333523083.

Hurnik, D. 2003. Barn Wash/Disinfection Trials, The Pig Site, http://www.thepigsite.com/articles/883/barn-wash-disinfection-trials/

Johan, V.K. and Arie, W. 2011. Pig farming in the tropics: From free range to small- scale intensive production systems. Agromisa Foundation and CTA, Wageningen

John M. King, Lois Roth-Johnson, David C. Dodd and Marion E. Newsom (2014). The Necropsy Book. A Guide for Veterinary Students, Residents, Clinicians, Pathologists, and Biological Researchers. Published by Cornell University, USA.

Knoesen, J.G., Aucock, H.W. & Gardner, M.H. Pig farming – General hints. Directorate Agricultural Engineering and Water Supply and Pig Health Scheme: SA Meat Board. Undated.

Kwamina, E.B., Josephine, NT. Kweku, A. and Emmanuel, K.D. 2014. Economic and Market Analysis of Swine Rearing and Pork Production in Ghana. Journal of life sciences Vol 8 (8): 700-708

Kyriazakis, I. 2006. Whittemore's science and practice of pig production (pp. 105-147). Oxford: Blackwell publishing.

Lee, Jasper S., et al. 1996. Introduction to Livestock and Poultry Production. Danville, Ill.: Interstate Publishers, Inc.

Malcolmson, R. W., Mastoris, S. The English Pig: A History, 1998, 192 pp., Hambledon, London, UK. ISBN: 1852851740.

Manual on meat inspection for developing countries http://www.fao.org/docrep/003/t0756e/T0756E01.htm

Marie Gramer, Kurt Rossow, Jerry Torrison, Martin Bergland, Jim Collins and Rod Frank (2005). A Guide to Porcine Sample Submission and Diagnostic Tests. Minnesota University Veterinary Diagnostic Laboratory. USA.

Martínez, J.E. 2009. The Rotation of Disinfectants Principle: True or False? Pharmaceutical Technology (33) http://www.pharmtech.com/rotation-disinfectants-principle-true-or-false?id=&sk=&date=&pageID=10

McDonnell and Russell 1999. Antiseptics and Disinfectants: Activity, Action and Resistance, Clinical Microbiology Reviews, Jan. 1999, p. 147–179

Murrell, K. Darwin, George T. Woods, and LeRoy G. Biehl. "Trichinosis." Pork Industry Handbook. PIH 103. Lafayette, Indiana.

Murtaugh, S.M et al. 2000. A Survey of disinfectant use in hospital pharmacy aseptic preparation areas, Pharmaceutical Journal 264:446-448.

Musukwa, M. N.; Basics in Quality Pig Feed Mixing. ISBN 9982-56-014-X, Zambia

Musukwa, M.N.; Feeding Pigs 2005. ISBN 9982-56-011-5, Zambia

Musukwa, M.N.; Pig Housing and Equipment. ISBN 9982-56-012-3, Zambia

MWPS. 1983. Swine Housing and Equipment Handbook. 4th ed. MWPS, Iowa State Univ., Ames, IA.

NPPC. 1996. Swine Care Handbook. Des Moines, IA.

NRC. 1981. Effects of Environment on Nutrient Requirements of Domestic Animals. Natl. Acad. Press, Washington, DC.

NRC. 1988. Nutrient Requirements of Swine. 9th rev. ed. Natl. Acad. Press, Washington, DC.

Paul C. Stromberg (2008). A Satellite Seminar on Descriptive Gross and Microscopic Veterinary Pathology In Necropsy, Surgical Biopsy And Certification Examinations. Delivered as pre-conference during the XXV Annual Convention of Indian Association of Veterinary Pathologists, held in at Indian Veterinary Research Institute (IVRI), India.

Perez, R.; Feeding Pigs in the Tropics, 1997, 185 pp., FAO, Rome. ISBN: 92-5-103924-0.

Pinilla, J. C., Geiger, J., Kummer, R., Piva, J., Schott, R., and Williams, N. H. (2008). Management strategies to maximize weaning weight. American Association of Swine Veterinarians 39th Annual Meeting Proceedings: 185–191.

Pinilla, J. C., Kummer, R., Piva, J., and Williams, N. H. 2006. Key components to wean 11+ piglets per farrowing. American Association of Swine Veterinarians 37th Annual Meeting Proceedings: 215–220.

Pork Issues Handbook. Des Moines: National Pork Producers Council, 1996/1997.

Research Institute for Pig Husbandry; Applied Research in Pig Husbandry in the Netherlands, 1991, 28 pp., Rosmalen: Research Institute for Pig Husbandry.

Sainsbury, D. 1972. Pig Housing. University of Cambridge, Farming Press Ltd., Ipswich.

Serres, H.; Manual of Pig Production in the Tropics, 1992, 262 pp., CAB International, Wallingford, UK. ISBN: 851987842.

Shannon, M.C. and Fangman, T.J. 2000. Swine Antibiotics and Feed Additives: Food Safety Considerations, M.U. Guide, G2353.

Stacy, S. and Tom, H. 2010. Local Effects of Hog Production on Farm and Non-Farm Economic Outcomes. Selected Paper prepared for presentation at the Agricultural &Applied Economics Association 2010 AAEA, CAES, & WAEA Joint Annual Meeting, Denver, Colorado, July 25-27, 2010.

Straw, B.E., D'Allaire S., Mengeling, W. L.; Diseases of Swine, 1999, 1256 pp., Blackwell Sciences, Oxford, UK. ISBN: 63205256.

Susanne Küker, Celine Faverjon, Lenz Furrer, John Berezowski, Horst Posthaus, Fabio Rinaldi and Flavie Vial (2018). The value of necropsy reports for animal health surveillance. BMC Veterinary Research 14:191.

Swine Care Handbook. Des Moines: National Pork Producers Council, 1996.

Taylor DJ. 1999. Pig Diseases. 7th Edition.

Taylor, Robert E., and Ralph Bogart. Scientific Farm Animal Production. 3rd Ed. New York: Macmillan Publishing, 1988.

Thawley, David G., Donald P. Gustafson, and Robert R. Ormiston. "Pseudorabies." Pork Industry Handbook. PIH-38. West Lafayette, Indiana: Purdue University Cooperative

Thornton, K. 1984. Practical pig production. Farming Press Ltd., Suffolk.

Thornton, K. 1988. Outdoor Pig Production. Farming Press Books, distributed in North American by Diamond Farm Enterprises, Alexandria Bay, NY.

Whittemore, C.T. The Science and Practice of Pig Production, 1998, 704 pp., Blackwell Sciences, Oxford, UK. ISBN: 0632 0500861.

Index